Disasters

Current Planning and Recent Experience

Mike Walsh
BA, POST. GRAD. CERT. ED., SRN,
ENB COURSE 199 (A&E), DIP.N

Senior Lecturer

Department of Nursing, Health and Applied Social Sciences
Bristol Polytechnic

Edward Arnold
A division of Hodder & Stoughton
LONDON MELBOURNE AUCKLAND

© 1989 Mike Walsh

First published in Great Britain 1989

British Library Cataloguing in Publication Data
Walsh, Mike, *1949–*
   Disaster: current planning and recent experience
   1. Great Britain. Disaster relief.
   Planning
   I. Title
   363.3'48'0941

   ISBN 0–340–48669–4

Whilst the advice and information in this book is believed to be true
and accurate at the date of going to press, neither the author nor the
publisher can accept any legal responsibility or liability for any errors or
omissions that may be made.

Typeset in Great Britain by Wearside Tradespools, Fulwell, Sunderland
Printed and bound in Great Britain for Edward Arnold, the
educational, academic and medical publishing division of Hodder and
Stoughton Limited, 41 Bedford Square, London WC1B 3DQ by
Biddles Ltd, Guildford and King's Lynn

Dedication

This book is dedicated to the survivors and their rescuers, and to the memory of those who were not so lucky.

Major incidents 1984–1988. The map (opposite) indicates locations as listed in the left-hand column.

Num-ber	Date	Location	Incident	Approx. no. of casualties*
1	24.01.84	Off Guernsey	Ship sinks, Radiant Mel	9; 16 dead
2	20.04.84	Heathrow Airport	Bombing	20; (5)
3	16.05.84	Liverpool St Station, London	Train crash	40; (5)
4	23.05.84	Abbeystead, Lancs	Explosion	30+; 17 dead; (4)
5	30.07.84	Falkirk, Scotland	Train crash	60+; 13 dead
6	12.10.84	Brighton, Sussex	Bombing	30; 5 dead
7	11.10.84	Wembley, London	Train crash	60+; 6 dead
8	24.11.84	Oxford Circus Underground, London	Fire	'many' evacuated; 15 hospital patients
9	04.12.84	Salford, Manchester	Train crash	77; 2 dead
10	11.12.84	M25, Surrey	Road crash	10+; 10 dead
11	14.03.85	Luton, Bedfordshire	Football riot	47; 31 arrests
12	11.05.85	Birmingham, West Midlands	Football riot	70; 1 dead
13	11.05.85	Bradford, Yorkshire	Fire	280 hospital patients; 53 dead
14	31.05.85	Battersea, London	Train crash	105; (14)
15	22.08.85	Manchester	Air crash	80 hospital patients; 55 dead; (15)
16	09.09.85 10.09.85	Handsworth, Birmingham	Riots	137 arrests; 2 dead
17	28.09.85 29.10.85	Brixton, London Brixton, London	Riots Riots	over 200 arrests and 50+ injuries
18	06.10.85	Tottenham, London	Riots	255 injured; 1 dead
19	21.10.85	M6, Preston	Road crash	27; 13 dead; (13)
20	07.11.85	Haywards Heath, Sussex	Train crash	50; (13)
21	24.12.85	Holborn Underground, London	Fire	200 evacuated; (1)
22	23.06.86	M4, Maidenhead	Road crash	13 dead
23	26.09.86	Beverley, Yorkshire	Train crash	39; 9 dead
24	11.09.86	Bristol, Avon	Riots	14; 75 arrests
25	19.09.86	Stafford	Train crash	76; 2 dead
26	06.03.87	Zeebrugge, Belgium	Ship sinks	402; 137 dead
27	19.08.87	Hungerford, Berkshire	Shooting	16 wounded; 16 dead
28	05.09.87	M6, Lancaster	Road crash	7; 8 dead
29	09.09.87	M4, Heathrow	Road crash	74; 4 dead
30	28.10.87	M61, Preston	Road crash	12 dead
31	08.11.87	Enniskillin, Northern Ireland	Bombing	60+; 11 dead
32	18.11.87	Kings Cross Underground, London	Fire	60+; 32 dead
33	07.07.88	Piper Alpha, North Sea	Fire	25+; 165 dead
34	20.08.88	Omagh, Northern Ireland	Bombing	29; 8 dead
35	12.12.88	Clapham, London	Train crash	115; 34 dead
36	21.12.88	Lockerbie, Scotland	Air crash	200 homeless; 270 dead

* Where known, number admitted to hospital in parenthesis.

The list is by no means exhaustive, being merely a summary of incidents. During this period there were the bitterly fought industrial disputes of the miners strike and the Wapping print works, the continual violence in Northern Ireland and many incidents involving football hooligans that did not make it on to the front pages of the national newspapers. Many such incidents must have stretched local emergency services to near disaster point as may many a serious road traffic accident not reported here. The table is based upon current news reports in *The Times*, therefore, casualty figures are approximate.

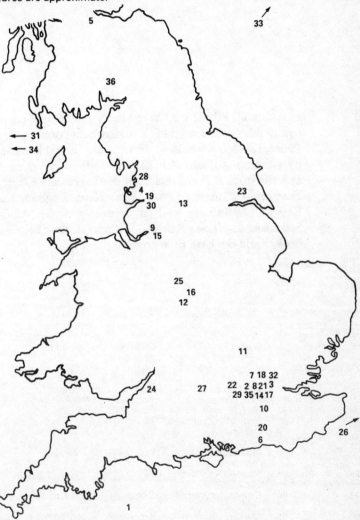

Map showing location of major incidents 1984–1988.

Acknowledgements

In addition to those who have kindly contributed chapters to this book, I would like to thank the Metropolitan Police, London Ambulance Service, the Central Electricity Generating Board (CEGB), the staff at Heysham A and Heysham B Power Stations, the Lancashire County Emergency Planning Office, BBC News London, the Regional Newsroom staff in Bristol, and also Annie Strickland and Tessa Rawlins. Without all their help the book would not have been possible.

Contents

	List of contributors	ix
1	Introduction: Why do we need disaster planning?	1
2	Immediate first aid for survivors	9
3	Injury associated with disaster	25
4	Multidisciplinary teamwork and communication	48
5	The mobile team	71
6	The role of the local authority emergency planning officer	86
7	The psychology of disaster	91
8	Disaster: the media and the emergency services	118

Case studies

9	Terrorism: the IRA bombing campaign in London, 1982/1983	131
10	A study of urban mob violence: the Tottenham riots, 1985	140
11	When an aeroplane catches fire: the Manchester International Airport disaster, 1985	150
12	A day at the football match: the Bradford City Football Club fire, 1985	161
13	The Abbeystead Pumping Station explosion, 1984	172
14	A motorway crash: the M6 disaster, 1985	181
15	Nuclear disaster planning after Chernobyl, 1986	186

Contents

16 A man and a gun: the Hungerford massacre, 1987 204

17 Conclusion: the future of disaster planning in the United Kingdom 211

Postscript: Lockerbie 216

Index 225

List of contributors

Anne Eggleton SRN formerly Head of Accident and Emergency Department at Princess Margaret Hospital, Swindon.

Mary N Haslum BSc, PhD, C.Psychol. is Principal Lecturer in Psychology at the Nursing, Health and Applied Social Sciences Department at Bristol Polytechnic.

Ian D Lee RGN, ONC, Acc. Cert is a Clinical Nursing Officer in the Accident and Orthopaedic Unit at Wythenshawe Hospital, Manchester. He has lectured on the organisation of Major Accident Planning throughout the country, and was on the planning team of Wythenshawe Hospital Major Accident Procedure.

Michael McColl FRCSI is the Consultant in charge of the Accident and Emergency Department at the Royal Preston Hospital.

Veronica Pickles RGN is Sister of the Accident and Emergency Department at the Royal Lancaster Infirmary.

Peter Salt RGN, RMN is Charge Nurse of the Accident and Emergency Department at Bristol Royal Infirmary. He is responsible for the Major Accident Planning for Bristol Royal Infirmary's Accident and Emergency Department and the Mobile Flying Squad.

Rodger Sleet MB, ChB, FRCP (Ed), FRCGP is a Consultant Physician and Director of Clinical Services of the Accident and Emergency Department at Southampton General Hospital.

Brenda Verity SEN, RGN is Sister of the Accident and Emergency Department at Bradford Royal Informary.

Stuart Westbrook RGN, ONC, REMT is Clinical Nurse Manager of the Orthopaedic Unit at the Royal Lancaster Infirmary.

1

Introduction: Why do we need disaster planning?

It will never happen to me will it? This is a common human defence mechanism employed whenever we think the unthinkable, and it can often be found when mention is made of disaster planning. Whether it be the busy accident and emergency (A&E) unit or ambulance personnel, fire or police services, they all have great demands on their time, so why should they be enthusiastic about planning for something that has never happened in their area? It will never happen here will it?

How could a modern ferry sink within yards of the harbour entrance in a matter of seconds? Who could imagine the London Underground or a football stand in a place like Bradford in Yorkshire turning into a blazing inferno? Who could have imagined rioting mobs shooting at the police and burning and looting their way through the streets of our cities, while terrorists sink to the depths of bombing a Remembrance Day parade? And let us not forget Michael Ryan and Hungerford.

These things could never have been imagined by most people, yet they happened, and it was the emergency services who had to deal with the carnage and human suffering left in their wake. We must therefore put aside the defence that it will never happen to us . . . it can.

Having accepted that disasters can happen, and like lightning they can strike in the same place twice, why are special plans needed? The answer lies in the simple definition of a disaster; 'a situation where the normal emergency services have been overwhelmed and can no longer cope'. Extra resources have to be mobilised and new unusual problems call for unusual solutions, new procedures are therefore required (but they should be as close as possible to standard working practices, more of this later). In short, a disaster plan is needed to be able to cope with this 'one off' set of circumstances.

It is not possible to give a more precise definition of a disaster than the one given above. Hospitals, in particular, seem prone to rigid definitions involving a fixed number of casualties before they will implement their disaster plan. The fallacy of this approach has been seen many times in A&E departments where one bad road traffic accident, perhaps coinciding with several seriously injured or ill patients already in the department, has stretched the unit to breaking point, yet, because only 10 people were involved, it has not been declared a disaster and the department has been denied the resources it needed. Hungerford produced 14 live casualties, not enough for a formal 'disaster', but consideration of the extent of the injuries suffered by the victims should suggest the need to move to a more flexible definition of a disaster, rather than simply counting heads.

The state of disaster planning varies widely in the United Kingdom (UK), but it is hoped that 1987, the 'Year of Disaster' as it has become known, will stimulate fresh planning and work. All areas have plans, but even the best of them can never be perfect. One of the best ways of improving plans is to learn from other people's experiences. This is the rationale for the second part of this book in which a range of different events that have occurred in the recent past in the UK are described.

As an introduction to the business of disaster planning, it is worth looking at certain key characteristics that mark out disasters as different from the day-to-day work of the emergency services. It is these characteristics that have to be built into our plans.

Unpredictability

It should be apparent that if disasters could be predicted they could be avoided. This then is the first problem that has to be faced. Clearly, it can be said that certain types of situations are more likely to produce major incidents, for example, busy motorways, and airports or areas where large crowds assemble such as football stadia or theatres, but it is only a probability, and there is little way of knowing *when* a disaster will strike. Then there are other situations which nobody could imagine might be dangerous such as a small market town in Berkshire on a summer's day (Hungerford), a pumping station in Lancashire (Abbeystead), or a Remembrance Day parade (Enniskillin).

There are two implications for planning here. In the first case, potential risk factors within the area should be identified, for example, a stretch of motorway, a large chemical plant, etc., and contingency planning carried out to at least ensure vital elements such as good access.

As an example, consider a stretch of motorway. If the accident happens on one carriageway, would it be easier to transport casualties to hospital A, but, if on the other carriageway, to hospital B? If so, there should be plans to ensure that the emergency vehicles arrive via the shortest route on the correct side of the motorway, facing the right direction for the speedy transport of casualties to the correct hospital.

Another example involves access to complicated sites such as a large chemical plant, a nuclear power station, or an underground transport system. Do the emergency services have plans showing clear access? Has there been full coordination, in advance, with security staff on site to ensure that precious time is not wasted arguing about access?

Advance planning which looks at possible sites of major disasters within the area covered by the emergency services is therefore crucial. Equally important is to consider the quality of radio communications within the area. Are there any notorious blackspots where because of local terrain or buildings communication is going to be difficult? If such areas are known, it is important to think of alternatives to get round the problem, especially if the area is near a potential disaster location.

When a disaster happens, whether it is at a risk location or not, there is unlikely to be any warning (except perhaps in the event of a natural disaster). Given this unpredictability, *plans must be simple and flexible*. It is impossible to try and anticipate every contingency and draw up detailed plans to cope with them. Neither can the plans be rigid as the situation will be unanticipated, changing rapidly, and the staff in the front line, whether that be in the field or the hospital A&E unit, must have the freedom to make the decisions they see fit in the circumstances. Delegation of authority to those staff most involved rather than rigid rules drawn up in a comfortable office light years away from the real situation is required.

Disaster plans should facilitate the work of the emergency staff

3

rather than get in their way. Flexibility and simplicity are therefore the key words.

Unfamiliarity

As previously discussed, a disaster situation tends to be very different from normal practice; this is one of the main reasons for needing specific plans. Given the strangeness of the situation and the great stresses that it will generate, it is clear that this is not the time to be expecting staff to learn a whole new set of procedures. In short, the nearer working practices can be to normal, the more efficiently they will tend to be carried out.

The plan should therefore, as far as possible, have staff performing their normal duties in their normal way. If staff are to function in a new environment, then every effort should have been made to give them some familiarity with their new role. A good example of this involves sending a mobile team from a hospital to the site. For medical and nursing staff this is a new experience and their effectiveness must be impaired by the alien surroundings. A sensible approach might be to have a rota of staff who make up the mobile team, sufficient in number so that there will always be enough staff available to respond immediately. This group of staff should then be given frequent training opportunities to familiarise themselves with the equipment set aside for the team. They should also familiarise themselves with conditions in the field by spending shifts with the ambulance service to gain some insight into the conditions that they might have to work in. It is not good enough to simply say that two doctors and two nurses will be taken off the wards to make up the mobile team! Apart from ensuring that they are of sufficient seniority and clinical experience to be of value, they must also be given the field training to familiarise them with the likely disaster environment.

Speed

Another characteristic of disasters in the UK is the speed with which they happen. Elsewhere in the world, natural disasters such as famine usually have some warning and may evolve over a period of months. The sort of man-made disasters with which we in the UK are familiar tend to have no warning and to be over very suddenly.

The implication of this is that a rapid response time is essential for any worthwhile plan. Not only does this emphasise the need for simplicity and flexibility, but it also opens up the vital area of communications. A log jam at the communications area can slow the responses of all the services and introduce confusion, frustration, and eventually chaos.

The suddenness and magnitude of a disaster is mirrored in the suddenness and magnitude of the communications that are generated. The systems must be able to handle this flood of messages quickly and reliably. Events can move so quickly that the first warning a hospital has of a disaster is the arrival of casualties at the A&E department brought in by well-meaning members of the public. The Birmingham pub bombings in 1974 were an example of this sort of phenomenon.

Environmental conditions

There are two aspects to consider here: firstly, where the environmental conditions are the backdrop to a man-made disaster and, secondly, where they are the disaster. In the first case, field teams may have to contend with fog, rain, and the cold, as well as working in the dark, surrounded by rubble and broken glass, and have further hazards to contend with such as unexploded bombs or leaking gas mains. This has implications for the clothing and equipment issued, in addition to how effective specialist medical teams may be under such conditions.

The second situation to be considered is the occurrence of a natural environmental disaster. Fortunately the UK does not possess active volcanoes, nor does it suffer from prolonged droughts or feel more than the occasional mild earth tremor. However, a once in a thousand year downpour can wipe out a village such as Lynmouth in Devon with frightening suddenness, while prolonged rain exacerbated perhaps by snowmelt may lead to extensive flooding of lowland areas for several days at a time. Can the emergency services in the low lying areas of major river systems, such as the Severn or Trent, cope with such a contingency? Those especially prone to danger are the elderly, particularly if they live alone and are dependent on community nursing services, meals on wheels or home aides to survive in their own homes. It is important that the health service and local authority social services departments consider how people in need may be identified and assisted in such situations. Prolonged severe winter weather brings with it a number of deaths from hypothermia, not just in the elderly, and may also be fitted within the framework of a disaster, as it produces problems that normal resources cannot cope with.

Is it possible that a hospital could be flooded out or isolated by flood waters for several days? Before hospital staff answer no, they ought to check with their local water authority and consider the probabilities of such an event. If necessary, could the basement and ground floor be evacuated? Could the essential utilities such as power and heating be maintained during a flood? Has the hospital got enough supplies in-house to survive being cut-off from the outside environment for several days?

In general, with natural disasters the timescale of events is much more drawn out, perhaps over several days. There should also be some sort of warning. However, the hurricane that struck the south east of England in October 1987 drew attention to the fact that, despite all the modern environmental monitoring systems, natural disasters can still happen without warning.

One major incident that has not occurred in the recent past, but which should be borne in mind as a possibility in considering the interface between man and nature, is that of a dam failure. Look upstream and ask what would be the effects of a sudden failure in any major dams in your area. It couldn't happen? That is what they said about the Titanic!

Why me?

Survivors of a disaster may suffer major psychological trauma if they have witnessed horrible scenes and maybe lost relatives and loved ones. The suddenness and unpredictability of it all leads inevitably to the question, 'Why me?'. Survivors will not be thinking and acting rationally and sensibly and they may have suffered far more psychological damage than physical, the effects of which will last for days, weeks and maybe the whole of the person's life. Planners should also remember that members of the emergency services are not immune from such stresses.

A feature of life in the 1980s has become the incidence of mass civil disturbances, whether in the form of street riots such as Tottenham, or the activities of football hooligans, hence casualties may also show a great deal of aggression. Consideration should be given to the persons to whom this anger and aggression is directed. Is it wise to allow the two parties to meet again or should plans be made to treat the two sides separately?

Multi service involvement

This is an inevitable aspect of disaster management; police, fire, ambulance and hospital services will all be involved, possibly together with the armed services and other public utilities such as local authorities, gas boards, railways, etc. All are very different organisations with different hierarchies and chains of command and responsibility, all talking different languages with different areas of expertise and priorities.

If rescue and recovery work is to be effective, all these different agencies are going to have to work together in a coordinated way. This means they need to be aware of each other's areas of responsibility and systems of working. Matters such as these cannot be left until the night, they have to be well thought through in advance and clearly understood by all concerned.

Comprehensive discussion and agreement in the planning stage is essential, but that is not all. There is little use in senior officers of the various agencies agreeing who is responsible for what if the staff on the ground do not know what has been agreed. There must be full communication down the chain of command and training opportunities so that the personnel on the ground know their roles and responsibilities.

Conclusion

From this overview, the following principles that are essential for good planning can be drawn up.

1   A disaster is a situation where normal resources can no longer cope.
2   Key words are simplicity and flexibility.
3   As far as possible, staff should follow familiar work patterns and procedures. Any major changes must be accompanied by adequate training.
4   The plan should be capable of a speedy response.

5 Maximum priority must be afforded to communications to ensure they are reliable and fast.

6 Possible disaster locations should be considered and factors such as access and communication considered in advance.

7 Environmental hazards should be considered in their own right, as well as the background to a man-made disaster.

8 Survivors will need intensive psychological support in addition to physical care. Rational behaviour cannot be expected.

9 The situation may be one in which there has been violent and bitter combat between two factions.

10 *There must be adequate preparation and planning between all the services involved, and the results of such work must be known to all grades of staff. Training and communication are the two words that matter here.*

11 It must be recognised that disaster can happen anywhere at anytime and, unlike lightning, it can strike twice in the same place. Continuous updating of plans incorporating lessons learnt from others is essential, together with a positive attitude that this is a worthwhile job that may one day save many people's lives. The efficiency of the operation mounted by Belgium's emergency services in the disaster at Zeebrugge involving *The Herald of Free Enterprise* roll-on/roll-off ferry is testimony to this.

2

Immediate first aid for survivors

Introduction

It is likely that the first rescuers on site will not be medically trained. The purpose of this chapter is therefore to describe simple but possibly life-saving steps that can be taken by anybody before ambulance crews or a hospital medical team arrive.

The patient's condition in these early minutes may be critical, although she/he may look deceptively well. The casualty staggering around covered in blood looks the most dramatic, but probably has the least serious injuries. It is the silent casualty, lying on the ground, who should be the first priority. Care must be started correctly, despite the fact that the conditions in which rescue personnel are forced to work will often be very difficult. It is essential therefore to keep interventions simple and practical.

Care of any casualty must be controlled by the priorities essential to maintain life, the so-called 'ABC' of resuscitation. This involves clearing and maintaining the airway (A), assisting the patient with breathing if needed (B), and ensuring there is an adequate circulation of blood around the body (C); airway, breathing, circulation, or ABC.

Airway

The first priority on reaching a casualty should be to check if they have a clear airway, if they are breathing, and whether they have a pulse. If conscious, our own airway is protected automatically by the closure of the passage into the lungs (the trachea) with the epiglottis. This means that food can be swallowed without any of it entering the trachea and blocking the passage of air into the lungs. Similarly, if a conscious person vomits, the epiglottis closes and protects the airway. In addition, the cough reflex will expel any foreign material from the back of the throat preventing it from threatening the airway (Fig. 2.1).

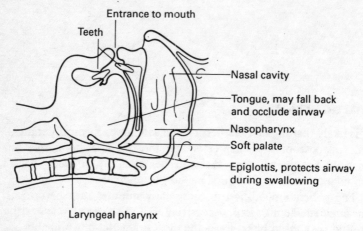

Fig. 2.1 The upper airway.

However, if a person is unconscious, all these defence mechanisms are lost with the result that any foreign material such as blood from facial injuries, vomit or water, may be inhaled into the airway and asphyxiate the casualty. In addition, if any unconscious person is lying flat on their back, the tongue may flop backwards and block the airway.

From this discussion, it can be seen that a casualty who is unconscious is at great risk due to the threat to their airway. They are top priority for evacuation and medical attention. However, due to the risk of making unknown injuries worse (e.g., neck injuries), unconscious casualties should not be moved unless they are in immediate danger. This should be left to the expert skills of the ambulance crew. In the meantime, vital steps can be taken to clear and maintain the airway by using fingers to clear the mouth of debris and to remove any false teeth.

The problem of the tongue flopping back and blocking the airway now has to be dealt with. To avoid this the jaw should be thrust forwards and the head tilted back, as shown in Fig. 2.2. The effect

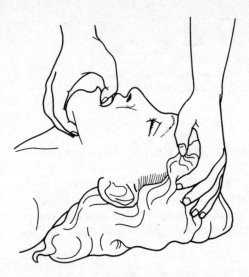

Fig. 2.2 Head tilt–jaw lift manoeuvre. The mandible is pulled forward using the thumb and forefingers.

of this manoeuvre is to lift the tongue clear of the airway and, as long as the patient's head is kept in this position, the airway will remain clear.

Even with these steps, if the patient is lying flat, vomiting will lead to a blocked airway as there is no way of removing the vomit before the patient inhales it. The correct step therefore is to turn the casualty gently into the recovery position (Fig. 2.3). Lying on the side in this way will allow vomit, blood, etc., to drain by gravity from the mouth rather than be inhaled, and it will also prevent the tongue from flopping backwards and blocking the airway. If possible, all unconscious patients should be put into this position as a preventative measure, rather than waiting for vomiting to occur.

There is one problem however, and that concerns the possibility of a serious neck injury. It should be assumed that an unconscious patient has a neck injury until proven otherwise. The danger is that movement of the neck could displace an unstable injury and cut the spinal cord resulting in permanent paralysis from the neck down, or death. It is partly because of this risk that unconscious patients should not be moved if at all possible. In placing the patient in the recovery position, great care should be taken to ensure that there is

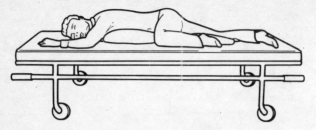

Fig. 2.3 Recovery position for unconscious patients.

no rotation or flexion of the neck. The whole trunk should be moved as one unit with the head, and neck supported at all times. In clearing the airway the emphasis should be on pushing the jaw forward to minimise neck movement rather than tilting the head back (Fig. 2.4).

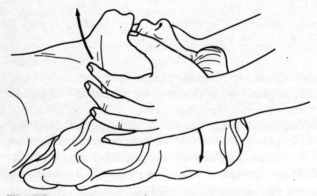

Fig. 2.4 Jaw thrust manoeuvre for clearing airway in an unconscious patient suspected of having cervical spine injury.

If the rescuer needs to perform 'mouth-to-mouth' resuscitation (see Fig. 2.5), the casualty should be placed on their back and the airway maintained with the head, tilt-jaw, thrust method described above.

Breathing

The importance of breathing to maintain life is obvious. If oxygenated blood does not reach the brain for a period of more than three

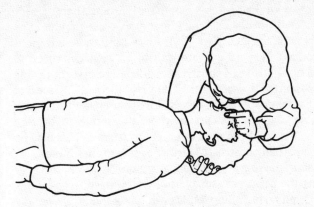

Fig. 2.5 Position for mouth-to-mouth resuscitation. Note head tilted back to clear airway and nostrils pinched closed.

minutes, permanent brain damage will develop which will rapidly become fatal. Fortunately the air that is normally exhaled by a rescuer contains sufficient oxygen to prevent brain damage occurring if it can be directed into the casualty's lungs; hence the effectiveness of 'mouth-to-mouth', or expired air resuscitation.

Having cleared the airway as described above, the rescuer should check the casualty's breathing by watching for chest movement or placing their ear close to the mouth to listen for any breathing sounds. If no breathing is detected, the rescuer should then place their mouth over the casualty's mouth and pinch their nostrils closed, take a deep breath and blow steadily into the casualty's mouth watching to see that the chest rises in response. If this does not happen the lungs have not been properly inflated. The most likely causes for this are that the rescuer did not blow hard enough, the airway was not properly clear (check the neck position), or that their mouth was not completely over the casualty's. This first breath should be followed by a second one immediately, and the casualty should be observed to see if they start breathing spontaneously.

If no respiratory effort is made, the rescuer should continue at a rate of 12 breaths per minute. It is very likely that the casualty will have no effective circulation either, their heart having stopped beating, and it will be essential to start this other basic life support function which is described in the next section.

If the casualty is a small child, it is possible to cover both the

13

mouth and nose with the rescuer's mouth and the aim should be for shorter more rapid breaths, at a rate of about 20 per minute. The rescuer can breathe for a casualty in this way until more advanced medical equipment and personnel are available. The golden rule is to never give up until medical help arrives as there are cases of people who had apparently drowned after being submerged in freezing water for half an hour still being successfully resuscitated.

It is possible that the casualty may be attempting to breathe spontaneously, but still be in need of urgent assistance. This may be due to either a partially obstructed airway or severe chest injury.

As discussed in the previous section, a completely blocked airway will mean that the casualty is unable to breathe at all; respirations will be absent, and no breathing sounds will be audible. If the airway is partly obstructed, the breathing is noisy. This is a cardinal sign that the casualty needs intervention to free the airway and allow normal breathing. Simple removal of the cause of the obstruction (e.g., false teeth) from the mouth as described in the previous section may be life-saving.

If the casualty has received a severe chest injury there may be bleeding into the pleura (the sac of tissue that surrounds the lungs) or air may be able to enter this space collapsing the lung underneath (pneumothorax). The casualty may have suffered fractures of the ribs. If a rib is fractured in one place, this will cause the victim severe pain, but if several ribs are each fractured in two places, the result is an unstable section of chest wall (known as a flail segment) that will severely threaten the person's ability to breathe at all. This injury will probably be accompanied by bleeding into the pleura and air also entering this space (haemopneumothorax). Finally there may be an open wound communicating directly with the lungs.

The effect of this range of possible injuries is to severely embarrass the casualty's ability to breathe to the point where it may rapidly prove fatal. A casualty with evidence of chest injury or difficulty in breathing is clearly a high priority for medical assistance and evacuation. The rescuer should assess how easily the person is breathing, whether they have chest pain, and if it is made worse by breathing. If the casualty is unconscious, a quick examination should be made of the chest wall to look for signs of bruising or marking. The pattern of the casualty's clothing may be tattooed into the skin after a severe blunt injury, or there may even be tyre marks across the chest. The two sides of the chest are also checked to make sure that they look the same and are moving together and equally on respiration.

Chest pain, coughing blood, noisy, laboured breathing, unequal movement of the two sides of the chest on breathing, skin tattooing or bruising, and the presence of a penetrating wound are all indications for high priority evacuation.

Whilst waiting for evacuation, the casualty should not lie flat, this will make breathing a great deal more difficult. If the person is able, they should be sat up at an angle of approximately 45 degrees, more upright still if they can tolerate it. Any wound should be covered immediately and if an unstable section of chest wall is suspected it should be splinted if possible. Lying the patient on their injured side will allow maximum expansion of the lung on the uninjured side and will tend to splint the injured side. The rescuer should remember when moving the casualty that chest injuries are very painful.

The casualty rescued from a fire also needs careful attention paid to their breathing. In the next chapter some of the noxious gases that are released when combustion takes place will be discussed. It should be noted here however that the smoke inhaled from a fire can cause serious damage to the lungs and airway. Upon rescue the casualty should be given oxygen, or at least got into the fresh air, and cared for in an upright position to assist breathing.

If the casualty has actually inhaled flame (as shown by burning and soot around the nose and mouth) the swelling that will develop in the upper airway associated with burnt tissue may rapidly block the airway leading to asphyxiation. Such a casualty is a high priority for evacuation.

Problems associated with the inhalation of toxic fumes and damage to the airway were a major concern in the Manchester International Airport fire described in Chapter 11, but less prominent in the Bradford City Football Club fire described in Chapter 12. The reason is probably associated with the fact that the Manchester victims were trapped *inside* a burning aircraft, while most of the Bradford casualties were in the semi-open air due to the fact that a football stand is open to the front and sides to permit visibility of the pitch.

Circulation

Breathing however is only half the battle for the patient, for it is to no avail if there is no effective circulation to carry oxygen to the brain and other vital organs. To check whether the heart is beating, the rescuer should feel for the carotid pulse in the neck (Fig. 2.6). If this is absent, it may be assumed that the heart has stopped and therefore resuscitation involves not only clearing the airway and breathing for the patient, but also working to restore a circulation.

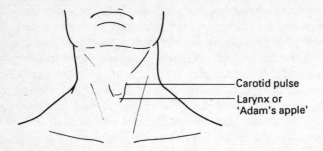

Carotid pulse

Larynx or 'Adam's apple'

Fig. 2.6 Location of carotid pulse.

Circulation is restored by external chest compression. The principle is to rhythmically compress the chest, thereby squeezing blood out of the large vessels and the heart around the circulation. If this is done effectively, in combination with 'mouth-to-mouth' or expired air resuscitation as described previously, brain damage is prevented and the patient's heart may start beating spontaneously. Whatever the outcome, the casualty is in the best possible condition when an advanced ambulance crew or medical team arrive, giving them the best chance of survival.

For effective chest compression, the rescuer should use both hands placed on the casualty's sternum (breast bone) just below half-way down (Fig. 2.7). If possible, the casualty should be lying flat on a solid surface and the rescuer should use about half their body weight to lean on the casualty's chest, depressing the sternum 3 to 4 cm (1.25 to 1.50 inches). The arms should be straight and the rescuer should use a rocking motion to steadily compress and release the chest wall.

A rate of 70 to 80 compressions per minute should be aimed for. In order to maintain this basic life-support, the rescuer should seek to establish a regular rhythm of 15 chest compressions to two breaths. This rate should be kept going as long as possible. The

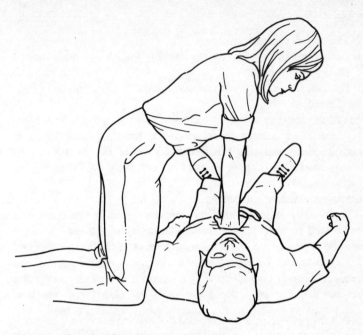

Fig. 2.7 Position for chest compression.

rescuer should not underestimate how tiring this can be and if assistance is available it should be utilised. If two people are performing cardiopulmonary resuscitation (CPR), one should concentrate on the breathing, while the other looks after chest compression, working at a rate of five compressions to one breath.

It is a ratio of 15 compressions to two breaths for solo CPR, and five to one for two person CPR. Periodically the rescuer should pause to check for any spontaneous signs of breathing or heart beat (check carotid pulse) as chest compression with a normally beating heart is dangerous.

If a young child is involved, it may be necessary to use only one hand for chest compression, and in the case of a baby, the thumbs of each hand will suffice. The rate should be correspondingly faster, about 100 times per minute.

One final point to be raised in connection with mouth-to-mouth resuscitation is the exaggerated fear of contracting AIDS. There is no medical evidence to suggest that it is possible to contract this disease from mouth-to-mouth contact.

Summary

1 Is the casualty conscious?
2 If not, is the airway clear, is the casualty breathing and is there a carotid pulse (ABC)?
3 If the casualty is not breathing spontaneously, the airway should be cleared.
4 Breathing for the casualty is commenced with two quick breaths.
5 If there is no carotid pulse, step 4 is followed with 15 chest compressions and continued with a ratio of two breaths to 15 compressions. If there is an assistant two person CPR is carried out at a ratio of five to one.
6 Summon assistance urgently.
7 The casualty is given artificial respiration until the rescuer is exhausted or until help arrives. The safety of the rescuer must also be remembered. At regular intervals the casualty is checked for spontaneous breathing or heart beat and the position of the rescuer's hands on the casualty's sternum is also checked. The rescuer's hands may slip away onto the chest wall which is dangerous as it reduces the efficiency of chest compression and may lead to fractured ribs.

Other aspects of first aid

Shock

This is a term much used in dealing with the survivors of disasters and smaller scale accidents. It is also a much misused and misunderstood term. In its strict medical sense, shock means a situation where a person's body tissues are not receiving enough oxygen. In other words, the circulation is not transporting oxygen around the body at the required rate. Shock is manifested by a pale skin, rapid pulse, low blood pressure and often deep, gulping respirations (air hunger). The casualty is also typically anxious and restless. If this condition is not quickly relieved, changes occur within the body that will lead to serious permanent damage (e.g., kidney failure) and eventually death.

The most likely cause of shock that will be encountered in disaster situations is blood loss from injuries (both internal and external) and also loss of plasma from the circulation due to burns. If the casualty has lost a litre of blood, or is suffering from burns affecting 20% or more of the body surface, shock will develop.

Estimating external blood loss is difficult and nearly impossible if the bleeding is internal. As a rule of thumb, try and envisage the mess made by dropping half a litre of milk, and compare the extent of the fluid to the blood loss from the casualty (0.50 of a litre is approximately a pint) (Fig. 2.8). Signs of pronounced swelling and bruising indicate internal blood loss, and it should be remembered that a fracture of the tibia (shin bone) results in the loss of half a litre of blood and a fracture of the femur (thigh bone) at least one litre. If there are penetrating injuries (e.g., gunshot wounds), or crush injuries (e.g., falling masonry), the development of shock is highly likely.

The rescuer should be able to recognise the signs of shock if they are present in a casualty, and also be aware of the sort of injuries that will lead to the development of shock in the near future, even if the casualty is not manifesting such signs at present. Shock casualties need immediate medical treatment if they are to survive and should be given a suitable priority for evacuation to ensure they get the life-saving care needed from either ambulance personnel or the mobile medical team.

There are important steps that the rescuer can take while awaiting the arrival of medical assistance. Firstly, any obvious bleeding can be stopped by direct pressure to the wound. A tourniquet should never be used to control bleeding, it is not necessary and will cause damage to the rest of the limb by depriving it of its blood supply. The patient should be laid flat with their legs elevated if possible; this improves the return of blood from the lower (less essential) part of the body to the vital heart–lung–brain system. Any fractures should be immobilised by splintage (see p. 23); this will reduce blood loss and relieve pain (pain is a potent factor in making shock worse). If oxygen is available it should be given to the patient to breathe. Finally, psychological support and reassurance will be very helpful, not only on humanitarian grounds, but also on good physiological grounds. Reducing stress and anxiety will tend to reduce the amount of pain that the casualty feels.

An important point here is that the patient must not be allowed to eat or drink anything. The reason is simple; they may well require immediate life-saving surgery under general anaesthetic. If the stomach contains food or liquid this will increase the hazards of the

(a)

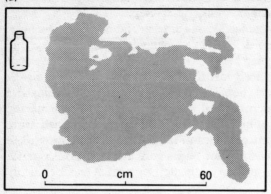

(b)

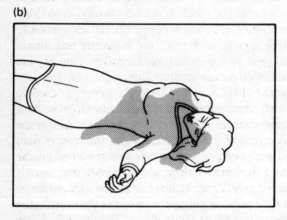

Fig. 2.8 Bloodshed **(a)** 0.50 litres (1 pint) on an unabsorbent surface makes a pool of about 60 cm (2 ft) square. **(b)** 0.25 litres (0.50 pint) will soak a dress right through and leave a considerable amount of blood on the surface beneath it.

anaesthetic due to the possibility of the patient vomiting. The traditional hot cup of sweet tea or tot of alcohol, beloved of outdated first aid manuals, has no place in modern rescue and first aid work. Keep the casualty nil by mouth at all times.

It should be remembered that the sort of shock that being referred to here is a physical condition, rather than the psychological shock produced by being involved in a disaster. Chapter 7 explores the psychological condition of disaster survivors in some depth.

Wounds and fractures

The importance of stopping bleeding has been discussed in the previous section. A word of caution is needed here as it is possible that a rescuer may concentrate on the obvious bleeding to the exclusion of a more immediately life threatening condition such as an obstructed airway. Assessment of the casualty is their airway, then breathing and circulation (ABC) before starting to look for wounds and fractures.

Bleeding

Wounds are dealt with by direct pressure. The temptation to remove any objects that are projecting from a wound should be resisted. Such material should only be removed under the controlled conditions of an operating theatre because of the following unknowns; depth of the wound, any vital structures that may be involved, and the effect of removal (e.g., a catastrophic bleed).

It must be repeated that tourniquets should never be used to control bleeding, only direct pressure. This can be applied by a rescuer pressing firmly over the wound (or the casualty if able) or the application of a dressing and pressure bandage. If the rescuer does not have a first aid kit available, improvisation is the order of the day. When applying a pressure bandage, always ensure that there is a normal circulation beyond the bandage. Normal circulation is checked by feeling for a pulse or noting the colour of the skin. In the heat of the moment it may be applied too tightly, effectively becoming a tourniquet, and depriving the rest of the limb of its blood supply.

One further obvious advantage of a dressing is that it prevents further contamination of the wound. Even if no sterile dressing is available, a clean covering will help a great deal. Clingfilm, for example, provides an excellent improvised dressing for burns and other large surface abrasions which are not bleeding heavily, although its use will be limited if there is heavy bleeding. The covering of wounds has beneficial psychological effects not only for the casualty but also for other survivors.

Fractures and serious joint injuries such as dislocation occur in

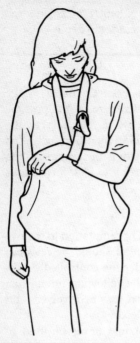

Fig. 2.9 Improvised sling using a belt to support an injured arm or shoulder.

situations where the casualty has been exposed to a considerable degree of violence (e.g., high-speed transit accidents or explosions). The nature of the disaster should therefore alert the rescuer to the possibility of such injuries amongst the survivors.

The classic sign of a fracture is localised bony tenderness. In other words, if the fracture site is pressed (gently), it is painful for the patient. However, the patient may be unconscious or very drowsy and confused. Other key signs to look for therefore are swelling, deformity and loss of function of the limbs. Pain may be expected to be present, but if the casualty is unconscious or moribund they will be unable to draw the rescuer's attention to any painful injury (see p. 9). Severe injuries may have bone protruding from the wound.

The correct first aid care of wounds and fractures/dislocations will help relieve pain, delay the onset of shock, and reduce fear and anxiety. In addition to these general effects on the patient, the healing of injuries locally without complications will also assist. The

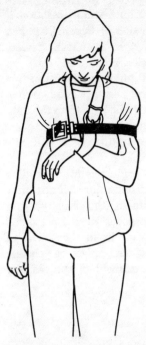

Fig. 2.10 An injury to the upper arm or shoulder may be further stabilised by splinting against the chest as shown here.

basic principle in dealing with suspected fractures is to immobilise the limb. This has the immediate effect of stopping the bone ends moving within the limb, causing pain and damage to other tissues such as nerves, blood vessels and muscle.

If the casualty is trapped by a limb and cannot be readily evacuated, amputation as a means of rescue may be considered. The prognosis for such a major procedure performed under field conditions is very poor and it should be considered as the last resort.

Immobilisation of an injured leg is simply carried out by strapping the two legs together, using the sound limb as a splint for the injured one. Any convenient material may be used for strapping (e.g., a belt). Padding should always be inserted to protect the bony prominences on the inside of the ankles and knees. Using the same principle, an injured arm should be supported with an improvised sling (Fig. 2.9) and if possible secured by strapping to the side of the body

(Fig. 2.10). Slings are usually triangular, but if improvisation is necessary folding any rectangular piece of material diagonally in half will make a triangle. Alternatively, a belt looped around the back of the casualty's neck and wrist will help support an injured arm.

Injured limbs will rapidly swell, and an important aspect of first aid is to remove any constrictions. This will permit a good circulation in the limb and prevent the patient suffering pain from the tight constricting effect of whatever is causing the problem (e.g., a bracelet or ring). If not removed immediately, the object will only have to be cut off later.

If the rescue worker follows the basic principles of controlling bleeding with direct pressure and immobilising injured limbs, they will have made a major contribution to reducing the casualty's pain and improving their long-term survival prospects. Rescue personnel should initiate such action as delays may occur in the arrival of ambulance personnel or the mobile medical team, given the chaotic nature of a disaster scene. The sooner treatment of the casualty begins, the better the prognosis.

Injury associated with disaster

In this chapter some types of injuries and conditions that are not commonly encountered by ambulance personnel or hospital accident units in day-to-day practice, but which may occur in disaster situations, are described.

Blast injury

The source of a blast may either be a deliberately detonated bomb or an accidental build-up of explosive material such as methane gas, as happened in the Abbeystead disaster. The body may be affected in several ways which can be summarised as follows.

1 A high-pressure blast wave moving radially outwards from the explosion.
2 The person may be physically thrown through the air by the blast wave, suffering injury upon impact with walls, floor, etc.
3 Burns from the explosion flash and also from fire which may develop amongst the wreckage.
4 The impact of material thrown through the air by the explosion, causing both penetrating and non-penetrating injury.
5 Crush injury from collapse of the building.

The effectiveness of debris in causing injury is revealed by the fact that in war time more than 80% of all injuries are caused by fragments from explosive devices (Owen-Smith, 1985). This fact is not lost on terrorist organisations such as the Irish Republican Army (IRA) who have packed their own bombs with materials such as nails and ball bearings to enhance their anti-personnel effects. As fragments from explosions are not streamlined, they rapidly slow down in their flight through the air. While they start out as high velocity particles, they soon become low velocity in nature. The significance of this will be explained later (p. 35).

An explosion creates a rapidly expanding body of gas that compresses the air around the bomb. This area of compression moves away from the explosion and may involve momentary pressures of thousands of pounds per square inch. On moving through the human body the blast wave will cause damage to hollow, air filled organs, mainly the lungs and eardrums, although the bowel may also be affected. Underwater explosions are much more likely to cause damage to the bowel than atmospheric explosions.

If the explosion occurs in a confined space, the situation is complicated by the effect of walls reflecting the blast wave in the same way that a mirror reflects light. The casualties may therefore be exposed to several pressure waves of varying intensity, rather than the single blast wave experienced in an open environment. This makes it very difficult to predict the seriousness of casualties based purely on distance from the explosion. Figures 3.1, 3.2 and 3.3 illustrate the location of casualties in three pub bombings carried out by the IRA and shows how unpredictable the distribution of casualties becomes in confined spaces.

It is possible for a casualty to have escaped direct injury from flying debris (they may have been behind a solid object that afforded protection) and therefore appear unmarked. However, the blast wave may have inflicted serious lung damage due to the dramatic changes in pressure that have occurred within the chest. This may be on a large scale associated with the sudden compression and recoil of elastic tissue within the lungs, and on a microscopic scale due to disruption of the walls of the alveoli. Such casualties may experience serious breathing difficulties in the next few hours as they develop pulmonary oedema and haemorrhage within the alveoli in response to the trauma their lungs have suffered (a build up of fluid in the lungs that interferes with oxygen–carbon dioxide exchange). This

---

3.1 (a) The Tavern in the Town public house, Birmingham. The position of people immediately before the explosion is shown with an assessment of the severity of injuries received. Eight of the dead could not be placed. The centre of the explosion is shown in the bottom right hand corner of the figure. **(b)** The Tavern in the Town public house, Birmingham. The incidence of eardrum rupture and of other auditory disturbances in the occupants of the bar following the explosion. Redrawn from Cooper *et al.* (1983).

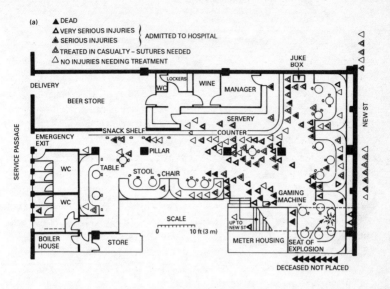

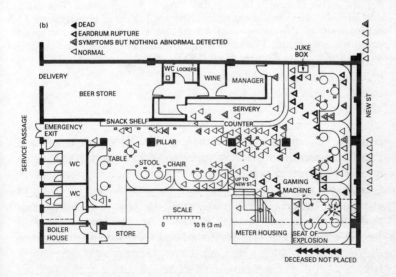

27

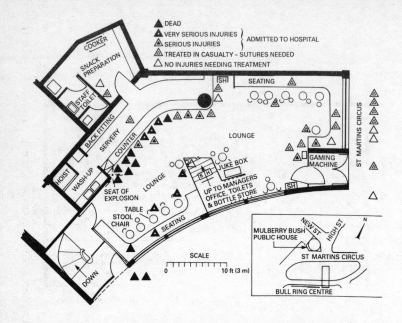

Fig. 3.2 The Mulberry Bush public house, Birmingham. The position of people immediately before the explosion is shown with an assessment of the severity of injuries received. Two of the dead could not be placed. The centre of the explosion is marked centre-left. Redrawn from Cooper *et al.* (1983).

condition is referred to as *blast lung*. Evacuation to hospital is therefore essential for all blast survivors, even if they have escaped injury from flying debris.

Intensive respiratory support may be required for survivors of explosions. Coppel (1976) has documented a series of 569 admissions to the Royal Victoria Hospital, Belfast, after bombings in Northern Ireland between 1971–75. He found that 68 required admission to the Respiratory Intensive Care Unit; 15 developed respiratory failure, five of whom were identified as suffering principally from blast lung.

These bombs contained low energy home-made explosives which

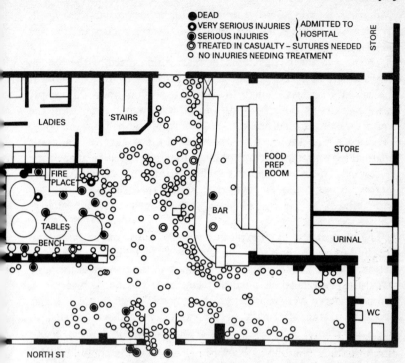

Fig. 3.3 The Horse and Groom public house, Guildford. The position of people immediately before the explosion is shown with an assessment of the severity of injuries received. A scale is not available for this plan. Some of the tables have been removed for clarity. The centre of the explosion was at the far left centre of the alcove containing the fireplace. Redrawn from Cooper *et al.* (1983).

meant that the casualty had to be close to the explosion to suffer a high enough blast pressure to develop blast lung. This explains the low incidence of blast lung in this particular series. However, with terrorist organisations becoming more sophisticated and gaining access to high energy military explosives, there is a prospect of any future intensive bombing campaign producing more blast lung casualties than the Belfast series of the 1970s.

One further effect of such a blast wave is that survivors will probably be deafened due to perforation of the eardrums. Tinnitus, a buzzing sound, is also common after an explosion. However, spontaneous healing of the ruptured eardrums occurs in the vast majority of casualties.

The next factor to consider is the blast wind caused by the sudden displacement of a large volume of air in response to the explosion. If the casualty is close enough to a large explosion, they will simply cease to exist as their body disintegrates. Moving away from the source, the effect is sufficient to remove whole limbs from the body. Experience has shown that casualties do not survive traumatic bilateral leg amputation, even though they may be alive at the time of rescue. The blast wind is capable of throwing casualties many metres through the air with the result that their injuries are compounded by the risk of being thrown against objects such as walls or debris.

The blast effects of an explosion will also cause major damage to any buildings, leading to crush injuries from falling masonry and debris. Rescue workers will be very aware of the danger of unstable structures, but hospital medical teams may not be so aware and should proceed very cautiously. Fragments of glass are a major problem in the aftermath of an explosion. Hospital teams in particular should therefore be very careful, especially with regard to footwear; ordinary shoes will be of little use when scrambling over glass strewn rubble. Caution should also be exercised due to consequent hazards from severed gas mains and electrical wiring which may still be live.

The effects of blast are much worse in a confined space due to the crushing effect of falling masonry, etc., the large supply of material that will be blown across the room by the blast, and the greater risk of a casualty being blown against hard objects. Experience with terrorist bombs has shown that leg and pelvic injuries predominate as the device is usually left at ground level. Owen-Smith (1985) has pointed out that in explosions occurring in confined spaces, approximately 25% of dead or seriously injured casualties have suffered traumatic amputations.

The energy of the explosion turns much of the room contents into projectiles capable of inflicting serious or fatal injury. Particles such as splintered wood, glass, and furniture fragments, are in addition to the casing of the bomb and any anti-personnel shrapnel packed into the device. Objects entering the body may or may not pass through, depending upon how much energy they possess and how much is deposited in body tissue. Other objects may cause injury on impact without penetration.

Cooper *et al.*, (1983) have shown that the most common injury pattern produced by relatively small explosions in confined spaces is superficial. Casualties have bruises, lacerations, and small missile entry holes in the skin, and often a characteristic tattooing pattern from dust particles driven into the skin. To give some idea of the extent of injury, one patient had 300 small pieces of wood removed from their body after the Tower of London bombing in 1974.

Looking at penetrating injury, an analysis of Northern Ireland bombings revealed that of bomb blast fatalities, 25% had suffered one or multiple penetrating injuries to the thorax, and 26% penetrating injury to the abdomen.

It is worth repeating the advice in the previous chapter concerning objects which are driven into the body of a survivor by the bast wind; leave the objects well alone even though they may be as large as the leg of a table. Whatever the size, removal should only take place under the controlled conditions of a general anaesthetic and an operating theatre.

The pulse of heat released in an explosion is capable of producing significant flash burns. However, clothing has been shown to afford good protection. Exposed skin such as the hands and face is usually affected, and the legs of female casualties wearing skirts are also at risk. The burns are usually superficial, but may be very painful and distressing, especially if the build up of facial oedema leads to the eyes becoming closed, causing loss of vision. There is of course the risk of secondary burns due to fire, especially with disrupted gas supplies and electricity cables in the proximity of highly inflammable materials such as modern plastics.

The effects of bomb explosions may be summarised in Table 3.1 which describes casualties from six major bombings (The Old Bailey 1973, Tower of London 1974, Birmingham pub bombings 1974, Guildford pub bombings 1974).

Crush syndrome

It is possible that a casualty may be trapped by wreckage, fallen masonry, rocks, etc., for a period of several hours before their release is possible. This brings with it the risk of developing what has been described as the crush syndrome.

31

Table 3.1 Effects of bomb explosions from six major bombings (from Cooper *et al.*, 1983).

Total number of casualties	385
Fatalities	28
Admitted to hospital	104
Wound types	
serious soft tissue damage or loss	56
burns	43
fractures	36
eye damage	13
blast lung	5
eardrum rupture	38

Damage to muscle by the material trapping and crushing the limb will lead to the release of a substance known as myoglobin which will enter the general circulation and cause renal failure. Many other serious systemic effects are possible including septicaemia (Jones, 1984). Therefore, the crush syndrome is potentially a fatal condition. In addition, there will be major soft tissue swelling which may lead to such high pressures within the limb that the blood supply is seriously reduced, leading to the risk of gangrene and the eventual loss of the limb.

A good account of a typical case was given by Jones (1984) in describing the effects of a rock fall in a Cornish tin mine. Two men were trapped 470 metres (1400 feet) underground, one of whom died shortly before rescue. The survivor, a previously healthy 30 year old, was eventually rescued after several hours with both legs and his left arm trapped by the rockfall.

The survivor was taken to a local hospital where an intravenous infusion was set up to stabilise his condition and he was then transferred to a major A&E unit. His left leg was swollen and tense, there was no voluntary movement below the knee, and the foot was blue and cold. However, X-rays revealed no bony injury. When a urinary catheter was passed, 400 ml of dark coloured urine was obtained containing myoglobin.

It was 26 hours after the accident before the patient was taken to the operating theatre for a fasciotomy, an operation involving dividing the tissues of the leg to try and relieve the pressure on the vital arteries and nerves. The surgeons found pale, lifeless muscle and, as no circulation could be restored to the limb, they proceeded to amputate the whole leg. This was necessary as the limb would now be of no further use to the patient and would only pose a threat to his life due to the development of gangrene, septicaemia, renal failure and various other complications of the crush syndrome.

The patient however went into renal failure and had to receive dialysis for a period of 19 days before fortunately his kidneys did revert to normal function and he was able to make a long but eventual recovery. It is worth noting that two of the victims of the Moorgate Underground disaster in London in 1975 died from crush syndrome.

Jones (1984) concludes that if a trapped limb has pulses at its extremities (i.e., distally) and appears viable, every effort should be made to rescue the patient with the limb intact as it can be saved. If the limb is cold, swollen, pulseless, and has no sensation or voluntary movement, urgent fasciotomy is essential to attempt to restore circulation. If circulation is not restored, as in the case discussed here, immediate amputation is needed to save the patient's life.

Bearing this in mind, the conclusion of Bentley and Jeffreys (1968) that a limb should only be amputated in the field if it is the only way a casualty can be extricated from wreckage should be remembered. Such a procedure in the field is a major life threatening event and should only be undertaken when the probabilities of survival without amputation have reached a very low point.

Chest injury

Given that the chest contains the vital heart–lung system, major injury constitutes a life threatening event. In an earlier section, the effect of blast on the lungs has been described (see p. 26). Other mechanisms of injury are possible, i.e., a blunt closed injury, or a penetrating wound with the object responsible possibly still imbedded in the body.

Apart from damage to major blood vessels and the heart itself, the most likely major complication facing the patient will be a pneumothorax and/or haemothorax. To understand these rather forbidding names, it should be remembered that the lungs are contained in a double walled sac called the pleura. If air or blood gets into the space between the two walls of the pleura, the effect is to collapse the lung underneath making it increasingly difficult for the patient to breathe properly. The presence of air in this space is called pneumothorax, likewise, blood in the pleura is known as haemothroax.

A pneumothorax and/or haemothorax may be compounded by a series of double fractures of the ribs, leaving several ribs each fractured in two places. This free-hanging section of chest wall is known as a flail segment and moves independently from the rest of the chest wall, seriously impeding respiration. Injuries such as haemothorax and/or pneumothorax may be life threatening unless the blood or air is removed from the pleura quickly via a closed chest drainage system. A one-way valve such as the Heimlich valve may be employed in field situations. This allows drainage of air and blood from the pleura, but does not permit air to enter the pleura from outside. The chest wall may need stabilising if a flail segment is present and breathing may need to be taken over for the patient with the use of an Ambubag (a hand powered ventilation bag) or ventilator. Walsh (1985), and Walsh and Eddolls (1988) have given full accounts of the problems presented by such injuries and their immediate management in the field and A&E unit.

The high priority that must be given to chest injury victims, be they penetrating or closed injury, can be seen from the fact that in World War I, 65% of victims died. However, this figure was greatly reduced by the introduction of a policy of management by closed chest drainage as the first line of management to remove blood and air from the pleura. Operative intervention does not automatically follow, i.e., thoracotomy, even if there is a penetrating injury. This may at first sight appear a little odd, but the fact that such a policy led to a reduction to 8% mortality in World War II, and 7.6% in the Vietnam War, speaks for the efficacy of this approach to major chest injury in mass casualty situations (Suleman and Rasoul, 1985).

Suleman and Rasoul (1985) have described a series of 150 serious chest injuries amongst battle casualties in the Iraq army. The subjects all survived evacuation from the battlefield to a major thoracic surgical unit. They found that 7% were closed injuries and that of the remaining 93% with wounds 83% were due to shell fragments and only 10% to bullets. The effectiveness of shrapnel in causing casualties is a lesson well learnt by the IRA, along with the various armed services of the world, hence the development of fragmentation munitions as a recent trend. The IRA bombs used in London in 1982/1983 (see Chapter 9) were crudely effective attempts at applying this fragmentation principle as they were packed with nails and similar material. Future bombs seem likely to contain a greater number of smaller particles.

Table 3.2 gives some idea of the frequency of occurrence of different types of chest injury when dealing with the effects of explosives outdoors. The table reflects injury distribution among 150 surviving battlefield casualties from the Iran–Iraq war (Suleman and Rasoul, 1985).

Table 3.2 Frequency of occurrence of different types of chest injury.

Injury	No. of casualties
Haemothorax	81
Pneumothorax	37
Chest wall only	20
Lung contusion/laceration	20
Perforation of diaphragm	17
Flail chest	12
Cardiac tamponade	4
Myocardial laceration	2
Injury of great vessels	2
Shock lung	2
Oesophageal injury	2

The total adds up to over 150 as some casualties had more than one type of injury. Of the 150 casualties, 99 were managed by closed chest drainage only, while 25 required surgery, and a further 3 needed tracheostomy. The remainder were managed conservatively, i.e., without chest drainage or surgery. The final mortality rate was only 3.3%, i.e., 5 casualties died, all due to hypovolaemic shock caused by major bleeding after battlefield evacuation. Experience in Vietnam showed there was a far greater survival rate with wound affecting the right side of the chest than the central and left central portions, i.e., adjacent to the heart and major blood vessels such as the aorta and pulmonary arteries.

High velocity bullets and other missiles

For our purposes, the definition of high velocity is a velocity greater than that of sound (344 m/sec; 1100 feet/sec). Rifles fire a bullet greater than this speed, while a handgun has a typical muzzle velocity of 220–330 m/sec (700–1000 feet/sec). For comparison, a

Colt Armalite 5.56 mm has a velocity of 1015 m/sec (3250 feet/sec) which is similar to the Russian AK74. The energy a bullet possesses increases with the square of its velocity. Double the velocity and you quadruple the energy and hence the destructive potential. Add to this the fact that the bullet is travelling faster than the speed of sound, which leads to the development of a shock wave ahead of the projectile and a subatmospheric pressure behind, it can be seen why such projectiles are so destructive and have to be considered in a class of their own.

When such an object enters the body, the effect is to momentarily generate a large cavity many times the bullet's size as tissue is thrust away from the object. Due to the low pressure zone following behind the object, the body tissue then collapses violently back on itself, sucking large scale contamination into the wound from outside the body. Elastic recoil takes place and several waves of expansion and contraction occur. The net effect is a large volume of destroyed body tissue and a grossly contaminated, deep penetrating wound. The denser the tissue, the worse the damage, thus muscle and dense organs such as the liver will be severely damaged, and bone may be shattered even though the object does not actually make contact.

Such gross internal injury may be concealed by the fact that the entry and exit wounds are very small. The presence of any bullet wound indicates a high priority for the medical team, in terms of setting up an intravenous infusion (IVI) as a precaution against shock and evacuating the casualty to hospital for emergency surgery. If it is known that a rifle was used, this is crucial information for the surgical team as it will completely modify the principles of treatment. High velocity wounds of soft tissue must be radically excised and then left open for several days before delayed closure of the wound takes place due to the very high risk of gangrene developing in the aftermath of the gross tissue destruction and contamination that will have occurred.

It is also unwise to attempt to guess what internal structures may be affected by simply drawing a straight line from the entry wound to the exit wound. Bullets are notoriously unpredictable in their path through the body, especially the lighter weight, high velocity rifle bullets that are being considered here. The use of explosive bullets is not impossible, and such projectiles will clearly inflict massive injuries on the victim.

If emergency personnel are unfortunate enough to be caught up in crossfire, as happened at Hungerford, they should remember that the range and penetrating power of modern rifles is awesome. A handgun is only effective at ranges of below 100 metres (300 feet), whether it be an automatic or a revolver. However, a rifle will inflict major trauma at ranges of up to 1000 metres (over half a mile away). Bullets from such weapons are capable of going straight through a parked vehicle or ambulance, so while sheltering behind a vehicle may hide you from a gunman's vision, it will not stop a bullet. The only part of a typical civilian vehicle with sufficient stopping power to afford protection is the engine block, so if possible shelter behind the engine and at all times stay low.

Burns and inhalation injury

Paramedical teams will be familiar with the treatment of burns from day-to-day trauma practice. A few observations are relevant here however when dealing with large numbers of burn victims.

Cold water is the most effective first aid treatment, it limits the burn damage and gives a great deal of pain relief. Blisters should be left intact as the fluid underneath is sterile. Infection is one of the biggest problems with burns. The severity of the burn will be increased if hot material is left in contact with the skin. Therefore, clothing which is smouldering should be removed if it cannot be soaked in cold water. Similarly, material such as hot pitch or tar which is adhering to the skin should be flooded with cold water. Apart from these exceptions, burnt clothing is best left on the patient so that it may be removed in the sterile environment of a hospital after the patient has had the benefit of powerful painkilling drugs.

Casualties involved in explosions may suffer flash burns to exposed parts of the body, typically hands and face. These burns are usually partial thickness and require hospital treatment. Oedema (tissue swelling) associated with such burns may make it impossible for the casualty to open their eyes with the result that they may think they have been blinded in the explosion. It is necessary to use tact and reassurance to the effect that the problem is probably due to swelling of the facial tissues and that after a few days it should resolve leaving the person with normal vision once they can open their eyes again. However, be cautious how such information is phrased as the casualty may indeed have suffered serious eye damage.

The chart in Fig. 3.4 shows the well known Wallace Rule of 9 method of assessing burn area (superficial redness or erythema is excluded from the calculation). Any burn covering 20% or more of the body surface must have an IVI and be evacuated to hospital urgently due to the risks of shock in addition to the severe hazard of infection. It should be noted that in assessing priorities for treatment

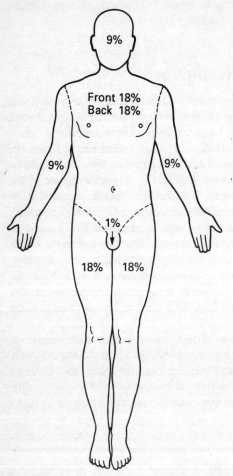

Fig. 3.4 Wallace's rule of 9 for estimating area of burns.

and evacuation, burns in excess of 65% of the body surface are not survivable; the insult to the body is too great. It is therefore suggested that, providing adequate pain relief has been given with intravenous analgesia, other patients may be evacuated ahead of patients with such major burns.

The most immediate hazard the casualty faces from burns is to their airway. If flames have been inhaled, as shown by soot in the nose or mouth, and the absence of the hairs normally inside the nose (these will have been burnt off), the patient is at great risk of occluding their airway due to burn oedema inside the respiratory tract. Such a person is a high priority for evacuation.

Many of the substances used in modern furnishings give off toxic fumes which on inhalation will severely affect the patient's respiratory tract. In addition, there is also the risk of asphyxiation from inhaling carbon monoxide and other products of combustion.

Budassi and Barber (1984) point out that plastic wall and floor coverings and telephone cable insulation cables contain polyvinyl chloride which on burning will liberate hydrogen chloride and phosgene, which are highly toxic and irritant gases. Combustion of polyurethane foam, used extensively in upholstery, will release hydrogen cyanide, while laquered wood veneer and wallpaper give off a variety of toxic fumes such as formaldehyde and acetaldehyde. The lung damage caused by these toxic fumes may not be apparent until 24 hours later when severe pulmonary oedema begins to develop. Consequently, any casualties evacuated from a smoke filled building should be evacuated to hospital even if their breathing appears to have quickly returned to normal. Any casualty with respiratory distress should be given oxygen and cared for in an upright position, rather than lying flat. This will greatly assist their breathing.

Emergency teams must leave the rescue of casualties from smoke filled buildings to the experts, the fire brigade, who will have the necessary breathing apparatus and experience, otherwise they may well become casualties themselves. Experience has shown that it is usually the smoke and fumes that cause most of the casualties, rather than the flames. For this reason, if rescue workers have the misfortune to be involved in an incident at a burning building, they are strongly advised to stay as low as possible as the hot gases and smoke will tend to rise towards the ceiling.

Carbon monoxide combines with haemoglobin in the blood

stream. Normally haemoglobin combines with oxygen and thus oxygen is transported around the body. However, carbon monoxide effectively crowds out the oxygen by combining more readily with haemoglobin, resulting in a dramatic fall in the blood's oxygen-carrying ability. Drowsiness, dizzyness and weakness are the early signs of carbon monoxide poisoning before the casualty lapses into a coma. Severe brain damage may develop before death finally occurs. A misleading sign with carbon monoxide poisoning is the pinkness of the skin, there is no cyanosis (a bluish-purple discoloration of the skin and mucous membranes) which is usually associated with respiratory failure. The pulse is strong and bounding while the blood pressure is elevated and pupils dilated. The casualty needs urgent oxygen therapy if there is to be any chance of resuscitation, and even then there may be permanent brain damage.

Methane (marsh gas or North Sea gas as it is known) is non toxic in itself, but in high concentrations will cause death by asphyxiation. The main danger is that when mixed with air (5% to 15% methane) it forms an extremely explosive combination, as many mining disasters bear tragic testimony, and latterly, the pumping house at Abbeystead in Lancashire. Burning in a good air supply methane forms carbon dioxide (as in your kitchen gas cooker), but burning in a poor air supply it forms carbon monoxide with potentially tragic consequences.

Riot control agents

The 1980s in Britain have been marked by the emergence of outbreaks of widescale civil disorder in urban areas. Disaster planning therefore needs to consider the effects of certain agents that may be used by the police and security forces.

Tear gas (Mace or CN) produces a feeling of heat and stinging on exposed skin and in the nose, excess salivation, and obscures the victim's vision due to the copious production of tears. The symptoms are distressing but in general not harmful, though they may last for several days. Vale and Meredith (1985) note that deaths have been reported from inhalation of tear gas when it has been used in confined spaces, while Cooper (1974) has described cases of severe eye damage. Casualties should be allowed plenty of fresh air and the eyes and exposed skin should be well irrigated with water to minimise the effects of the gas.

CS gas irritates the eyes and respiratory tract. Within 30 seconds of exposure there is a feeling of burning and tightness within the chest, followed by coughing, sneezing and a burning pain in the eyes. CS gas may trigger acute episodes of illness in people with long-standing lung disease such as bronchitis while, less commonly, disturbances in taste, nausea, diarrhoea, headaches and lethargy may occur.

Fresh air will help the casualties a great deal so they should be moved upwind of an area that has had CS gas canisters fired into it. As with tear gas, water should be used to irrigate the eyes and areas of exposed skin.

Radiation casualties

Radiation is all around us, light and heat are examples, and mostly it is of no harm. However, certain types of radiation are dangerous as they possess sufficient energy to disrupt the atomic structure of the material they encounter. Such radiation is known as ionising radiation and, as far as the human body is concerned, the basic problem is that ionising radiation interferes with the DNA in the cell nucleus, leading to abnormal cell division at low doses (causing the development of cancer), while at high doses the whole cell is killed. Logically it is the most rapidly dividing cells that are most readily affected, which explains why the blood cells are the most prone, leading to leukaemia at low doses and the wholesale destruction of the essential blood cells at higher doses.

The terms contaminated and irradiated need careful definition as they easily become confused. A person who is contaminated has radioactive material about their person, either externally on their clothing, skin, etc., or internally by virtue of it being swallowed or inhaled. They are therefore still emitting radiation, i.e., are radioactive, and possibly harmful to rescue workers as well as suffering increasing radiation injury themselves. A person who has been irradiated however is of no danger as they do not have any radioactive material about their person. They have been exposed to radiation which has done its damage to the person's body, but has then passed through.

In addition to suffering radiation injury, the casualty may also have suffered conventional injury. Due to the effects of radiation in preventing normal cell division, the effects of injury are made much

41

worse by radiation exposure, as the body's normal mechanisms of repair and defence against infection are severely handicapped. A further consideration is that the casualty may think they have been exposed to radiation when in fact they have not; this may lead to anxiety and fear. Unfortunately there is no immediate way of knowing if a casualty has been irradiated, you cannot see or smell radiation!

The amount of energy possessed by radiation used to be measured in rads, it is now measured in Gray (Gy). Differing types of radiation have different effects on the body, depending on the nature of the radiation (see Table 3.4). This is taken into account by another unit, the rem, which principally measures radiation energy but allows for differing types of radiation within any dose. The new unit to measure this effect is the Sievert (Sv). In practice, 1 rem may be taken as equivalent to 1 rad, therefore 1 Sv is approximately equivalent to 1 Gy. Table 3.3 summarises the different units used.

Table 3.3 Units used in radiation measurement.

1000 Microsievert (μSv)	= 1 Millisievert (mSv)
1000 Millisievert (mSv)	= 1 Sivert (Sv)
100 Rems	= 1 Sievert
1000 Microgray (μGy)	= 1 Milligray (mGy)
1000 Milligray (mGy)	= 1 Gray (Gy)
100 Rads	= 1 Gray (Gy)

A simple model of the atom describes it as a nucleus surrounded by orbiting electrons. The nucleus consists of positively charged particles called protons, and particles with no charge, neutrons. The electrons that orbit this central nucleus are less than 1/20000th of the mass of protons and neutrons, and carry a negative charge.

This structure is held together by various forces, normally in a stable configuration. However, some forms of certain elements (known as radioactive isotopes) are unstable and will decay at varying rates, emitting subatomic particles and energy. This is what is meant by the term a radioactive isotope. One further term worth defining is half life; this refers to the time it takes for one half of any given mass of a radioactive isotope to decay. It varies from fractions of a second to millions of years, depending on the isotope. ·

With these ideas in mind, some commonly encountered types of radiation are shown in Table 3.4.

Table 3.4 Differing types of radiation.

Type	Nature of radiation	Penetrating power Air	Body tissue
α ray	Stream of particles, each of which is 2 protons and 2 neutrons	6 cm	<1 mm
β ray	Stream of electrons	5 m	<2 cm
X-ray	Energy released by electrons changing position within atom	10–100 m	Whole body
γ ray	Energy released by nuclear particles changing configuration	>100 m	Whole body
neutron	Stream of neutron particles	>100 m	Whole body

Table 3.5 shows the effects of exposure to radiation, from the minimal permitted annual doses up to the large doses that may be involved in an accident.

The basic effect of radiation interfering with cell division has been described above. At low doses this has the effect of giving rise to increased risks of cancer, the available evidence suggesting the risk is directly related to the dose, i.e., twice the dose, twice the risk. It should also be remembered that a radiation linked cancer may not appear for many years exposure. At higher doses the effect of radiation on the body is much more immediate and is referred to as the radiation sickness syndrome. There is an initial reaction of nausea and malaise followed by a latent period when the casualty feels better, but then the full impact of the exposure strikes home as radiation effects take their toll on the body. The shorter the latent period the worse the prognosis.

The most reliable guide to a patient's exposure involves frequent monitoring of their white blood cell levels. Only by such observation over a period of time in hospital will the damage start to become clear. For emergency criteria, see p. 44 for a discussion of the Chernobyl radiation casualties. The implication is that all persons involved in a radiation accident should be transported to hospital for detailed screening and observation, even if they appear to have suffered no physical injury.

Monitoring of casualties for contamination will be carried out by site staff at an installation such as a Central Electricity Generating Board (CEGB) nuclear power station. If an incident has happened

Table 3.5 Effects of exposure to radiation (from BMA report 1983; Dace, 1987).

250 microsievert (μSv)	Average annual dose received by a member of the general public as a result of medical X-rays
1.4 millisievert (mSv)	Average dose per year to radiation workers from occupational exposure
2 mSv	Approximate annual dose from natural sources
5 mSv	Maximum permitted dose to a member of the public in the UK
10 mSv	If one million people received this dose, there would be 125 extra fatal cancers amongst that group (ICRP estimates)
50 mSv	Maximum permitted dose for UK radiation workers
0.1 to 1.5 Sv	Milder forms of radiation sickness with feelings of nausea and malaise, significant fall in white blood cell count above 0.5 Sv
1.5 to 4 Sv	Full bone marrow disease. Days 1–2 nausea, vomiting and malaise. Weeks 2–3 fever, mouth ulcers, skin haemorrhages. Loss of hair >3 Sv. Marked fall in blood count, maximum bone marrow depression at 30 days
4 to 10 Sv	As above plus serious disease of the bowel. Profuse bloody diarrhoea and loss of gut lining in weeks 1–2. At 4–4.5 Sv 50% mortality, at 6 Sv survival very unlikely
10 Sv plus	Central nervous system affected, lethargy, convulsions, coma and death within days
40 Sv	Death within hours

outside a site used to handling radioactive materials, the National Arrangements for Incidents Involving Radioactivity (NAIR) scheme exists (see p. 53). The NAIR scheme is a two stage call out system that will allow the police to get immediate advice about an accident involving radioactive material and, if needed, speedy access to the necessary monitoring personnel and expertise on scene.

If a casualty is contaminated, they may readily be decontaminated by being undressed and exposed areas of skin and hair washed with plenty of water. The water used will now be radioactive and therefore should be stored rather than allowed to run off into natural drainage channels or the sewer system. Decontamination may be carried out in the field if the patient's condition does not indicate the need for immediate hospitalisation. If a special decontamination unit is not available, inflatable containers similar to children's paddling pools may be used to collect the water, and, in fact, hospital A&E units should seriously consider purchasing toddler's inflatable pools for precisely this reason.

The CEGB will be responsible for handling and disposing of contaminated clothing, equipment and water in the aftermath of an accident involving radioactive material.

Decontamination should be carried out as quickly as possible to minimise the radiation injury to the casualty and the rescue personnel. However, in the event of the casualty requiring urgent treatment or resuscitation, this should take priority over decontamination. Resuscitation first, decontaminate second should be the order of events, otherwise a decontaminated corpse would be the result.

Protective clothing will not prevent radiation from passing through and irradiating personnel who are wearing it. Even the lead aprons worn in hospital X-ray units offer no protection against gamma rays. However, by preventing the wearer's clothes from becoming contaminated with radioactive material, protective clothing does serve a worthwhile function, providing it is removed and stored safely at the first possible opportunity.

Personnel may protect themselves from the harmful effects of radiation in several other ways. Firstly they should remember that radiation follows the inverse square law. This means that if you double the distance from the source of the radiation you reduce the intensity to one quarter of its previous level. Treble the distance and the intensity falls to one ninth of its previous level. Distance is therefore a valuable means of protection. Keep as far away as possible!

The second simple law of radiation protection concerns time – if exposed to a given level of radiation for twice as long, it has twice the damaging effect on the body. If required to operate in a contaminated area, work as quickly as possible.

If an incident has taken place at a nuclear power station, there may be a substantial amount of radioactive release in the form of gas or very fine particulate matter. Respirators may therefore be required to prevent inhalation of the material. Great care should always be paid to which way the wind is blowing and the instructions of on site monitors should always be followed. This applies with equal validity in the more likely case of an accident involving the release of toxic gases from a chemical works or tanker.

Protection from radiation may also be gained behind solid material such as concrete or brickwork, as this will absorb significant amounts, depending on the nature of the radiation (see Table 3.4). The suggestions to use distance, time and concrete or brickwork as defences against radiation exposure may seem rather obvious, but they are nonetheless valid.

Further safety steps include the use of badges which measure the total dose of radiation to which their wearer has been exposed. Such badges are worn routinely, for example, by staff in X-ray and radiotherapy units. In the event of an accident involving radiation, rescue personnel should wear the badges they are given as this will permit a reliable estimate to be made of the amount of radiation that they have been exposed to which is important for their own safety and long-term follow up. For their own safety, personnel should be guided by the instructions of on site monitoring staff at all times.

If an accident involves a nuclear reactor or nuclear waste, a radioactive isotope of iodine may be released. The body concentrates iodine in the thyroid gland leading to a build up of this radioactive isotope and, in the long-term, cancer of the thyroid. To protect staff from this risk, nuclear power plants stock iodine tablets which should be taken in the event of an accident. The body will preferentially concentrate this stable form of iodine in the thyroid, to the exclusion of the unstable, radioactive isotope, thereby greatly reducing the risk of cancer in the long-term. Rescue personnel should therefore be sure to take the iodine tablet which they should be offered in such a situation (see p. 197).

Fear of radiation, like a fear of anything that is potentially fatal, is not a bad thing. However, at times over the last decade or so there has been a tendency for this to be bordering on the hysterical and irrational. Emergency personnel are professional staff who should have a healthy respect for any hazard, but they should tackle a radiation emergency in the same logical and professional way as any other.

References

Bentley, G., and Jeffreys, T. E. (1968). The crush syndrome in miners. *Journal of Bone and Joint Surgery*, 588.

British Medical Association. (1983). *The Medical Effects of Nuclear War.* John Wiley, Chichester.

Budassi, S., and Barber, J. (1984). *Emergency Care.* C. V. Mosby Co., St Louis, USA.

Cooper, P. (1974). *Poisoning by Drugs and Chemicals.* Alchemist Publications, London.

Cooper, G. J., Maynard, R. L., Cross, N. L., and Hill, J. E. (1983). Casualties from terrorist bombings. *Journal of Trauma,* **23(11)**, 955–67.

Coppel, D. L. (1976). Blast injury of the lungs. *British Journal of Surgery,* **63**, 735–7.

Dace, M. (1987). *Radiation and Health.* Medical Campaign Against Nuclear Weapons, London.

Jones, R. N. (1984). Crush syndrome in a Cornish tin miner. *Injury,* **15**, 282–3.

Owen-Smith, M. (1985). Wounds caused by the weapons of war. In *Wound Care,* S. Westaby (Ed). Heinemann, London.

Suleman, N. D., and Rasoul, H. A. (1985). War injuries of the chest. *Injury,* **16**, 382–4.

Vale, J. A., and Meredith, T. J. (1985). *A Concise Guide to the Management of Poisoning.* Churchill Livingstone, Edinburgh.

Walsh, M. H. (1985). *A&E Nursing: A New Approach.* Heinemann, London.

Walsh, M. H., and Eddolls, T. (1988). *Emergency: A Guide for Ambulance Personnel.* Heinemann, London.

4

Multidisciplinary teamwork and communication

Rodger Sleet

Fortunately, the incidence of disaster for most health authorities is rare, but the ever present threat requires contingency plans which will coordinate the work of rescue services and health and local authorities to provide efficient care of the injured, the protection of the community, and minimise the disruptive effect on transport systems and in industry.

The successful management of a major incident involves early reconnaissance of the site, establishment of good communication between rescue services and hospital, mobilisation of rescue, medical and local authority support services, first aid care of the injured, and transportation to prepared hospital facilities. This response depends upon an agreed plan of action, trained personnel, good communication, and a coordinated response between rescue, medical and other services. Action is initiated by the receipt of the original emergency call and involves many organisations such as fire, police and ambulance services and continues to involve health and local authorities, voluntary organisations and in special circumstances other services, for example, coastguard, mine and mountain rescue teams. As with any chain, the overall strength is equal only to the weakest link. It is essential that all emergency services required in the event of a major disaster should have a coordinated plan of action, an agreed call out procedure of personnel, and prepared action cards (see p. 65) for use by those staff. The plan, action cards and communication should be regularly tested by periodic training programmes for all personnel involved and should be exercised with other necessary services and modified in the light of experiences gained and deficiencies recognised in rehearsal and actual incident.

Individual services will develop their own plans of action within the limitation of their available manpower and financial resources.

Plans should be developed in cooperation with other rescue and health organisations to ensure the use of a common terminology, rescue procedures, agreed clinical priorities for the sorting of casualties for evacuation (triage, see page 72 for further discussion), treatment and standardisation of clothing, equipment, and identifying tabards for members of staff. Coordination of disaster plans and agreed communication procedures should ensure efficient action, minimising the threat to the life of the individual casualty, and should be beneficial to the safety of the community as a whole. The rescue services and the receiving A&E departments and hospital will each expect a professional response from other services in the event of an incident. The Department of Health has established guidelines for district health authorities regarding planning for a major incident which have been published in circulars HC (76) 52, HC (77) 1 and HC (85) 24. It is expected that each health authority will develop a coordinated plan of action for the district health authority, its receiving and support hospitals, and the ambulance service. These plans should be coordinated with the individual plans of the fire services, the police, local authorities and other agencies. Recent publicity in the media regarding incidents has led to a high expectation from the general public that health authorities and other involved agencies will be able to react promptly and efficiently in the event of a major disaster.

A mass casualty situation has four recognised phases:

1 The initial 999 telephone communication from witnesses at the site notifying the occurrence of the accident and requesting assistance.
2 The response of the rescue services to provide an immediate presence at the site for rescue and care of casualties and their prompt evacuation to hospital.
3 The reception, resuscitation, assessment, documentation and subsequent management of the critically injured or severely ill casualties at the designated receiving hospital.
4 The security of the site and subsequent investigation of the cause of the disaster.

Communication

Communication is the key to an effective response from rescue and health services in the event of accidents involving small or large

49

numbers of casualties. The 999 emergency telephone system available in the United Kingdom provides a means by which witnesses to an accident can rapidly communicate with the necessary rescue services. It is essential that the initial call includes information as to the nature of the accident, its location, estimated casualty numbers and, if possible, identified rescue problems. The call will be passed to the emergency service deemed appropriate from the information received; usually the police. The receiving emergency service will respond by initially dispatching a reconnaissance unit and will notify other relevant services. In some circumstances, the incident will initially involve industrial, mine, or airport emergency services before involving outside agencies. Occasionally a major accident may occur in the neighbourhood of the receiving hospital (e.g., the Bradford City Football Club fire) and there needs to be an agreed communication link for alerting both hospital and outside agencies after casualties arrive at the A&E department. After initial assessment of the accident site, the emergency services can institute a planned response by dispatching adequate vehicles, personnel and equipment to the site. At this stage, notifying the receiving hospital of the accident and of the possibility of casualties will allow the hospital to initiate its own plan of action, establish a hospital control team, alert the A&E department and necessary support services, without disrupting the routine work of the hospital until the casualty situation is clarified. In most instances, communication to the hospital will be by telephone link from local ambulance control, but in some instances hospitals have developed direct radio links with the ambulance service which can be utilised in these circumstances. Where patients arrive unheralded at hospital there must be agreed contingency plans to notify necessary hospital and rescue services.

The site

Action is coordinated by the senior police officer present, except in the event of fire where the responsibility is assumed by the senior fire officer. The police, fire and ambulance services have extensive experience in working together in accident situations of all magnitude and have developed plans for interservice cooperation in the event of a mass casualty situation which allows for a high degree of coordination.

The police service

The senior police officer has a number of essential roles which include the following.

1 Establishing radio communication links between the site and the control centre in police headquarters. Initially this can be achieved by police vehicles arriving at the site and later by a designated mobile communication centre.
2 To provide controlled, unobstructed entrance and exit for rescue services to the incident site and designate parking areas for loading of casualties and unloading of equipment.
3 To designate, with the senior ambulance officer, a suitable area for casualty sorting, immediate treatment and for subsequent evacuation of casualties, and, where necessary, request medical advice or assistance at the site.
4 Establish and supervise temporary mortuary facilities.
5 Advise on the need to evacuate surrounding inhabited areas where there is potential danger of fire or explosion, and to supervise the evacuated to accommodation designated by the local authority.
6 To provide protection at the site for casualties, rescue workers and others, and security for damaged and undamaged evacuated industrial and residential property.
7 Following the successful evacuation of casualties, be responsible for collating forensic and other investigations at the site of the incident and prepare reports to the coroner and other appropriate authorities.

In addition to their site activities, the police are responsible for establishing and manning a casualty information bureau which coordinates casualty information from the site and receiving hospital for release to enquiring relatives. There will be a need for the casualty information bureau telephone number to be broadcast to the general community through local radio and television services. Police officers will also be dispatched to the receiving hospital to provide liaison services between the hospital control team and police headquarters. These officers will be responsible for collating and updating casualty information prior to it being forwarded to the casualty information bureau. The accurate collection of such information is essential if relatives and press enquiries are to be satisfactorily and accurately answered by the bureau and the nominated police press officer (see p. 125). There is a recognised need for a police presence at the receiving hospital in the event of terrorist activity or civil disturbance for security purposes and the interviewing of casualties and other witnesses. Police activity within the hospital is dependent upon effective pre-planning between the two services with clear agreed objectives for police activities.

The fire service

The fire service has three major roles at the site of any accident.

1 Containment and extinguishing of fire at the site and subsequent investigation of its cause.
2 Advice to other members of the rescue services and receiving hospital on chemical, toxic or radiation hazards. The prevention of further contamination, and advice on decontamination procedures.
3 The rescue of trapped and injured persons and the provision of first aid treatment in association with ambulance and police services acting at the site. In the event of fire it is the senior fire officer at the site who will coordinate fire fighting activities and rescue operations and will advise police in the event of chemical, toxic or other contamination. The fire service will provide its own communication vehicle at the incident to provide a link between fire fighting headquarters and the services at site.

Fire headquarters will have access to computer stored information regarding potential toxic and other hazards at the involved industrial site or involved transport vehicles, and they will be able to utilise this information to the advantage of other members of the rescue services, local authority and receiving hospital. Advice will therefore be available as to the nature of the toxic agent, the health risks, methods of decontamination and treatment of affected patients. Decontamination of patients and rescue workers is restricted at site to the removing of outer contaminated clothing of patients and the washing off of protective clothing and equipment for fire fighters, with the subsequent collection of contaminated water in inflatable pools for later disposal. Decontamination procedures followed by the fire services use cold water sources and are unsuitable for the treatment of injured patients, particularly in wet or cold weather conditions. The ambulance and receiving hospitals will expect the fire service to provide early warning of contamination hazards to patients, ambulance vehicles and crew, and advise on decontamination procedures or provide relevant sources of information regarding chemical hazard from the manufacturer, transporter or other advisory agents. The receiving hospital will need to have its own plan of action and facilities to decontaminate patients on arrival.

In the event of an accident involving radioactive material, it will be either the police or fire officer on site who will institute the NAIR scheme. Such assistance is provided in two stages.

The first stage enables the police to call on a nominated experienced person to advise them on any action to be taken. This person is usually a designated member of the hospital medical physics department who is able to provide advice by telephone or by direct assessment at the site of the incident. They will not be expected to cope with incidents or control of contamination unless these incidents are very minor. Where the contamination is potentially beyond their capability to control, the police would advise on steps to be taken to protect the public from exposure to radiation by the creation of barriers to bar access to the site, and covering and containing the contaminated material to prevent spread.

The second stage of the NAIR plan would then be instituted, calling on assistance from such agencies as the United Kingdom Atomic Energy Authority, the Central Electricity Generating Board (CEGB), British Nuclear Fuels Limited (BNFL), or the Ministry of Defence (MOD).

The Police will expect the district health authority to maintain an on call rota of designated medical physicists and to devise an effective method of out of hours communication for recall. The medical physicist should have been involved in the designated receiving hospital's pre-planning of arrangements to receive and decontaminate and treat patients who have been contaminated with radioactive material, as well as providing guidelines on the collection and disposal of contaminated clothing and dressings, the cleansing of ambulance vehicles, and decontamination of staff.

The ambulance service

The ambulance service is experienced in working with the other two

major rescue services, fire and police, and also the district A&E
department. In the event of a major incident the service has the
following functions.

1   The dispatch of sufficient vehicles and crews to provide neces-
    sary first aid and immediate care to the victims of the accident
    and assist in the evacuation of casualties to an agreed casualty
    clearing point. After sorting, to evacuate the patients according
    to an agreed priority.
2   The senior ambulance officer on site will advise the police on all
    casualty evacuation and will request medical advice on site or the
    assistance of the mobile medical team from a designated hospital
    or General Practitioner Immediate Care Scheme (BASICS).
3   To establish communication from site to ambulance headquar-
    ters to update the ambulance control team and the receiving
    hospital of casualty numbers and activities at the site and request
    reinforcements of vehicles or personnel. This communication
    will initially be from ambulance vehicles or officers' cars acting at
    site, but within a short period of time a designated communica-
    tions vehicle should be supplied.
4   To provide and maintain a suitable store of necessary equipment
    and supplies at site, including dressings, splints and intravenous
    fluids.

Basically trained ambulance crews can provide effective first aid
care, including control of the patient's airway, assisted ventilation
with bag and mask techniques or automatic ventilating apparatus,
control of external haemorrhage, splintage of spinal and limb
injuries and the relief of pain with the use of Entonox.

The development of a national programme in extended training in
ambulance aid will mean that there will be an increasing number of
advanced trained ambulance personnel with additional skills relevant to the immediate care of the accident victim, including
advanced airway support with endotracheal intubation and ventilation, the correction of hypovolaemic shock by the intravenous
administration of crystalloid or colloid solutions, and, where indicated, the use of selected drugs for the control of pain and other
problems.

The magnitude of the incident and the severity of injuries may
require medical presence at site to assist the police and ambulance
services. There needs to be a pre-agreed plan for the provision of

such assistance and the identification of suitably trained personnel to be called upon. Medical presence at a major incident site falls into the following two categories.

1 The provision of a Site Medical Officer (SMO).
2 Provision of a mobile medical team of suitably trained and equipped doctors and nurses.

The role of the SMO is to assist and advise the senior police officer in matters regarding casualty care, triage (see p. 72) and evacuation, and the necessity for a medical team to work at site with other rescue services.

The SMO is usually a consultant member of staff of the designated receiving hospital. Many hospital plans utilise the service of a consultant anaesthetist or surgeon. Experience from rehearsal and actual incidents reveal there may be delay in providing a suitably qualified doctor and often the consultant identified would be better employed working at the hospital in their normal clinical role caring for arriving casualties. Alternative solutions would rely upon the senior ambulance officer present to carry out the duties of the SMO and in many instances their knowledge and training equip them to undertake this role, or alternatively a designated member of the local BASICS can fulfil the role and has the advantage of working normally alongside police, fire and ambulance in lesser roadside accidents.

Hospital mobile teams can originate from the designated hospital, support hospital or adjacent district hospital. Such flying squad services have as their immediate objective the resuscitation and immediate care of the severely injured or trapped casualty, and assisting the ambulance service in the sorting of casualties into priority groups for evacuation and transportation to hospital. To be effective the teams need to have both suitably qualified experienced medical and nursing staff, adequately equipped and clothed to work at the accident site, and to be covered by sufficient accident insurance provided by the Department of Health of Social Security (DHSS) or private insurance schemes.

Prompt mobilisation of such teams is essential if they are to be effective. For this reason many health authorities have looked to the BASICS operating within their health district to provide medical aid at a major accident site, leaving hospital staff to manage the critically injured patient and other casualties on arrival at the A&E department, and subsequently in the wards and theatres.

For those A&E departments who are regularly involved in the provision of roadside care, action at the site is merely an extension of their normal responsibilities. However, for many hospitals who provide only a little or occasional assistance to the ambulance services, the ability to assemble a suitably trained and experienced team for early dispatch to the site may prove difficult, and alternative methods of medical assistance from BASICS is a satisfactory alternative.

The role of the mobile team is:

1 To assist the ambulance service in the triage of patients for evacuation.
2 To provide immediate care, including resuscitation procedures.
3 To update the hospital control team medical director on casualty numbers and injuries and other special problems.
4 To accompany and supervise the care of critically injured patients during transportation to hospital.

In the event of operative surgical procedures being required at the site, it will be the responsibility of the medical director of the hospital control team to ensure the dispatch of an appropriately experienced surgeon and anaesthetist to work with the medical and ambulance teams already at the incident. The medical team may be required to remain at site to assist where dismemberment is required to extract dead bodies from entrapped positions, but such duties would be deferred until the acute requirements of the incident have been resolved.

As the rescue response gains momentum, the police will be able to assess the need for resources and the possible duration of the rescue activities. At this stage, there will be identified requirements for rotation of staff, to arrange catering and other support at site and utilise voluntary agencies such as the Women's Royal Voluntary Service (WRVS) who will have developed their own contingency plans and rehearsed them during exercises with both hospital and rescue services. The local authority would be required to have its own plan of action to assist the police if there is a need to evacuate surrounding residential property. Holding areas, temporary accommodation and billeting procedures will be required and a pre-arranged plan agreed with responsible officers nominated to assist the police in the event of such evacuation being necessary. Where large numbers of people have to be moved, local buses can be commandeered to ferry people from endangered areas to temporary accommodation in local schools, recreational halls or other sites. The use of such vehicles relieves the pressure on ambulance services (see Chapter 6).

Special sites such as caves, mines, and offshore maritime situations all require their own major incident plans, emphasising coordination of the relevant rescue services with the normal rescue and hospital facilities. Offshore incidents are coordinated by the regional harbour master or the senior officer commanding local naval establishments. Communication is central to successful search and rescue operations coordinating coastguard, lifeboat and fire services. Casualty evacuation from ships at sea requires careful control and organisation to avoid unnecessary dispersal of the injured along a wide area of coastline. Disembarkation points need to be identified in any maritime disaster plan. The plan also needs to include action to protect and provide safe navigational channels, prevention of collision at sea between rescue and other vessels, and subsequent containment of oil spillage to prevent the contamination of beaches and fishing areas.

Large public events, including air shows, sporting activities and political rallies, will require adequate planning to coordinate rescue and medical services in the event of a casualty situation arising.

A major incident is a matter of public interest and will be reported by the media. Press facilities will need to be arranged at an early stage of the incident and the senior police or fire officer at the site will usually liaise with his colleagues so that each service provides an experienced officer to assist at an established press information point. This information point should be the only place at the scene at which factual and statistical information will be released to the media, and, as far as possible, the same information will be made available at the same time for the fire, police and ambulance headquarters to release. The officer in charge of the press information point will advise representatives of the press and other agencies on how they may approach the incident in safety, of private properties affected, and opportunities to film. The primary concern of the rescue services will be the rescue and removal of casualties and to secure safe conditions at the site. After these have been achieved, the needs of press representatives to reach vantage points and to speak to survivors who have no objection to being approached should be arranged. The press will not be assisted to approach or photograph shocked or injured victims. The police will expect the press to respect the laws regarding trespassing and the right of owners of property to deny access. A detailed account of the role of the media in disaster situation is given in Chapter 8.

The hospital

The designated receiving hospital has an A&E department and supportive facilities necessary for the assessment and treatment of severely injured and critically ill patients. The hospital will have its own major incident plan which will have been developed in cooperation with all necessary outside agencies and other support hospitals within the health district.

The *major incident plan* is divided into two stages

Stage one is an automatic phase during which key departments and services are alerted of the occurrence of the incident. The hospital control team is then established, the available bed state is determined, and inpatients who are suitable for transfer to other care facilities or for discharge to the community are identified. During the alert phase, communication is maintained between the hospital control team and the incident site by direct radio link or ambulance headquarters.

Stage two is a discretionary phase decided by the hospital control team and aims to supplement existing staff, as required, with simultaneous reduction of routine work in wards, in theatres and outpatient departments according to a pre-planned sequence and only as required by the progression of the incident.

The dispatch of a mobile medical team or SMO will be decided by the medical member of the hospital control team and, on their discretion, dispatch may occur to the site during the first or second stage of the plan.

The plan will need to include details regarding the collation of all patient information at the end of the incident in order that the hospital's response can be analysed and modifications to the major incident plan made as a result of identified deficiencies during the course of the incident. The response of the A&E department and other key facilities is dependent upon a well rehearsed plan of action, informed key staff, and available departmental action cards, supported by a good communication system and a trained hospital control team working from prepared facilities.

The development of hospital major incident planning within the health district is the responsibility of the district manager who will usually delegate the detailed planning to a responsible assistant and a district planning team. The responsibility for the planning of the receiving hospital lies with the individual hospital unit manager and that unit's own planning team.

The role of the district manager is:

1 To ensure that the delegated receiving hospital and its A&E department have an adequate plan of action for use in the event of a major incident.
2 To ensure that there are adequate facilities for the care of casualties at the receiving hospital and at other support hospitals within the district.
3 To coordinate hospital, ambulance and community health resources. To negotiate mutual support between adjacent districts and provide adequate insurance for medical and nursing members of the hospital mobile team working at site, and facilities and financial support for regular rehearsal in all aspects of the district's hospital plan.
4 To liaise with the regional planning officer if there are problems with district cooperation or cross regional boundary problems.

The district manager will usually be advised by a district major incident planning team which meets at regular intervals with a formal agenda and recorded minutes.

The planning team should consist of:

1 The district manager or their designated representative.
2 Representatives from the designated receiving hospital and medical and nursing staff.
3 A member representing support hospitals.
4 A district ambulance representative.
5 A representative of community services.

The committee will have the power to coopt other members from the police, fire or other services. The value of this committee lies in its ability to coordinate district-wide response and to develop channels of support with adjacent districts. The plan of action for the acute management of patients lies with the manager of the receiving designated hospital. The manager will usually delegate planning to a unit team which consists of:

1 A consultant in charge of the A&E department.
2 Another hospital consultant, e.g., a consultant surgeon.
3 A senior nurse or nursing manager.
4 A representative of the hospital support services.
5 A member of the ambulance services.

Again, this committee will have the power to coopt other members as indicated and will be expected to have a formal agenda for meetings and to keep the necessary detailed minutes of each meeting. This committee will be responsible for the developing of the hospital major incident plan which should be circulated in draft form both to the district and unit managers and to senior medical staff for comment. The draft should then be modified in the light of comment, agreed and printed. The plan should then be widely circulated to key departments and staff. Ideally, the unit manager should ensure that seminars are held which educate staff on the objectives of the plan and their own role. Relevant extracts of the plan should be reproduced in staff handbooks issued to junior members on appointment. It will be necessary for the unit manager to obtain broad agreement from medical, nursing and support services on the principle that departments and services are responsible for the regular education of their staff in their role in the event of a major incident, and they should be responsible for the production and storage of their departmental action cards and regular rehearsal and audit.

The role of the regional health authority in major incident planning is usually delegated to the regional emergency planning officer who was initially appointed to oversee civil defence but whose role has now been modified to include all aspects of disaster planning. Their role is to coordinate planning within the health region and to develop, where necessary, the concept of mutual aid, not only between health districts and adjacent regions, but to coordinate health service activity with that of the local authority and other agencies.

The DHSS has published its guidelines regarding the health authority's response in a major incident and its requirements in disaster planning. Currently the DHSS does not regularly collate and report on major incidents occurring in the United Kingdom, offer analysis of lessons learned, or promote new ideas relating to health service practice in the event of a major incident occurring. Disasters in recent years have led to pressure for a central register of major incidents, a pooling of experience, and making available some lessons learned from each incident. Central to the hospital response is the *telephone communication system*. The training and preparation of relevant action cards is the responsibility of the telephone manager. Each telephonist needs to be fully informed of his or her role in the event of a major incident for immediate access to their action cards, and there should be a planned reinforcement of staff as indicated by the magnitude of the incident. It is easy for the hospital telephone exchange to become overloaded and for the alerting of necessary departments to be delayed if communication procedures have not been well thought-out in the planning stage. The hospital control team, A&E department and other key services may require their own external lines which bypass the hospital switchboard.

Unit action cards should include instruction of recall of any members of staff using outside lines within the hospital, and should have a recommended procedure that when any members of staff off hospital site are notified, that member of staff should notify, using his own private telephone, another member of staff in a cascade system, again reducing load on the telephone services. Action cards prepared by clinical services managers, consultants and nursing officers should include a planned sequence of staff mobilisation using private lines.

The hospital control team

This team is mobilised in the first phase of a major incident. The team should be housed in designated accommodation equipped with telephone communication with the rest of the hospital and outside agencies. There should be all the necessary secretarial support for the team, relevant action cards, and a patient flow chart identifying the progress of individual patients within the hospital care system at any particular point in time, as well as check lists for members of staff required to report in the alert phase and as the incident develops.

The team usually consists of a medical director, senior nursing officer or manager responsible for nursing services, and the senior manager for the hospital site. The responsibilities and roles of the team are as follows.

Medical director

1 Control of medical staff mobilisation and deployment throughout the hospital to ensure that the medical services are prepared for the reception and treatment of casualties.
2 Coordination of acute medical and surgical teams and radiology and laboratory services to meet the needs arising from the incident.
3 To dispatch suitably trained medical personnel to the incident at the request of site rescue services.
4 The curtailment and takeover of:
   (a) necessary outpatients facilities;
   (b) operating theatres;
   (c) patient admissions.
5 Coordination and control of additional medical staff from adjacent hospitals in the event of an overload situation developing.
6 Authorising the issue of casualty lists and press statements. The latter function being in liaison with the hospital and police press officers after the next of kin have been informed.

The nursing manager

1 Assumes the role of senior manager until the senior manager arrives at the control centre.
2 Responsibility for the management of nursing services during the major incident. These duties will include:
   (a) mobilisation and deployment of nursing staff for the following:
      (i) mobile team
      (ii) A&E department
      (iii) wards
      (iv) theatres
      (v) intensive care unit (ICU);
   (b) compilation of current empty bed states within the hospital;
   (c) the preparation with medical staff of a provisional list of patients suitable for transfer to other care facilities such as adjacent hospitals or discharge to the community.

The senior manager

Ensures that proper communications take place within the hospital and that supply services are made available to meet the needs of the incident. The supply services will need to include:

1 The provision of adequate clerical support to the mobile control team.
2 Transport arrangements for the mobile team if they are to be dispatched to the accident site.
3 Medical records (in conjunction with the medical records office).
4 Adequate portering services.
5 Security and traffic control within the hospital grounds and signposting.
6 Designating a colleague to handle public relations.
7 Support services as appropriate; telephones, linen, catering and cleaning.
8 Delegating other managerial staff for administrative duties as may be required.
9 Notification of the occurrence of the incident to the district unit general manager.
10 To provide accommodation and direct telephone lines for the police and ambulance liaison officers operating from the hospital control room and elsewhere in the hospital.

The senior manager should confirm with the hospital switchboard that the reception of all emergency admissions has been transferred to adjacent hospitals in the district or elsewhere in the region, and inform the ambulance service. They should ensure that the visual display unit in the hospital control room is regularly updated, the information contained collated and given to the medical, nursing and support services.

They should also consider the need for, and deployment of, staff as marshals to oversee patient movement within the A&E department, the hospital, and at any point from where patients may be discharged.

The senior manager should be prepared to mobilise the following where needed.

1 Interpreters.
2 Voluntary agents such as the hospital League of Friends and the

WRVS through the designated voluntary services coordinator.
3   The hospital photography service.

The hospital control team will expect the A&E department, receiving wards, theatres and other services to act from their prepared action cards during the course of the incident.

The clinical services manager will have prepared their own unit's response in a major incident, written action cards, arranged storage in identified positions, and have rehearsed their staff at regular intervals in their role in the event of a major incident. Communication procedures and methods of reinforcing and rotating staff in the event of an incident should have been tested.

The ambulance service will be expected to provide a liaison officer to work with the hospital control team and to provide a further official to work within the A&E department, assisting in the unloading and dispatch of ambulance vehicles. Police liaison officers will be appointed to work with the hospital control team and with medical records at points of patient admission and discharge from the hospital. Police liaison officers will collate casualty information for subsequent use by the casualty bureau and, if required, will have a security role. A coordinated plan of action between ambulance, police and hospital services should promote an effective sorting of casualties into priority groups for resuscitation, assessment, treatment and documentation, prior to transfer to wards, theatres and ICU, for discharge from the hospital with minimum delay and confusion.

Problems of language are minimised if there is an effective method of access to interpreters, and the plan should nominate a member of staff who will keep a prepared list of interpreters and the languages in which they are proficient, and telephone numbers for work and out of work hours.

Effective management of an incident depends upon a well-prepared plan whose objectives are known by all key staff. A plan which has been developed in cooperation with the rescue services and other agencies is supported by good communication and trained staff. The plan should take into consideration general and local hazards within the health district and have contingency arrangements for the care of casualties from civil disturbance. This should include arrangements for the security of casualties and those working at the incident site, and possible separation of participants, casualties, and police within the hospital to prevent disruptive behaviour within the A&E department and elsewhere in the hospital.

For the response to be effective, training and exercise is essential. Hospital staff, members of rescue services and other agencies are better equipped to deal with the problems arising from an incident and the resulting casualties if they are fully aware of what is involved overall. The district plans should give the overall picture of roles and health authority response. The hospital plan will give a detailed description of the roles of individual personnel. All staff involved in a major incident should have access to the district and hospital plan.

Action cards containing written instructions are essential for training and direction of individual response in an incident (Fig. 4.1). Cards should contain clear and concise instructions of the individuals' responsibilities and outline key communication procedures. The preparation of such cards lies with individual departmental managers and consultants, and these cards must be reviewed and revised at regular intervals. Personnel should be aware of the presence of action cards and where cards can be located in the event of a rehearsal or actual incident. A useful supplement to action cards are wall charts which outline departmental action in the event of a major incident, and the proposed patient flow system and communication procedures within the department. Being permanently on display these charts provide a useful, constant *aide-mémoire* to departmental staff (Fig. 4.2).

Staff identified to participate in major incident procedures have different levels of requirement for education and training. Senior administrative, nursing, and medical staff on long-term contracts require less frequent training than junior staff who often rotate through short periods of employment every six to twelve months.

Many of these junior staff are essential members of the acute hospital service in the event of a major incident. It is essential that there are methods of familiarising themselves with the overall hospital plan and their own specific roles. Handbooks issued on appointment can include sections regarding the major incident plan, but it is necessary to supplement this information with formal lectures and presentations in order that they may be conversant with their duties in the event of a major casualty situation occurring. They must be familiar with the site and content of their relevant action cards.

(a)

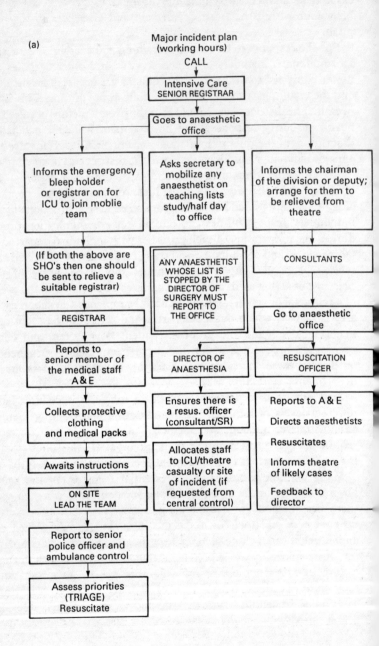

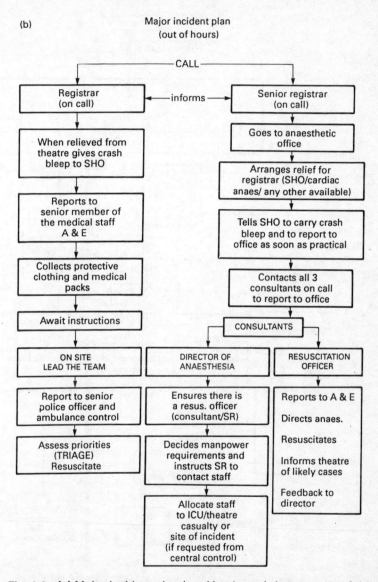

Fig. 4.1 **(a)** Major incident plan (working hours); by courtesy of the Shackleton Department of Anaesthetics, Southampton General Hospital. **(b)** Major incident plan (out of hours); by courtesy of the Accident and Emergency Department, Southampton General Hospital.

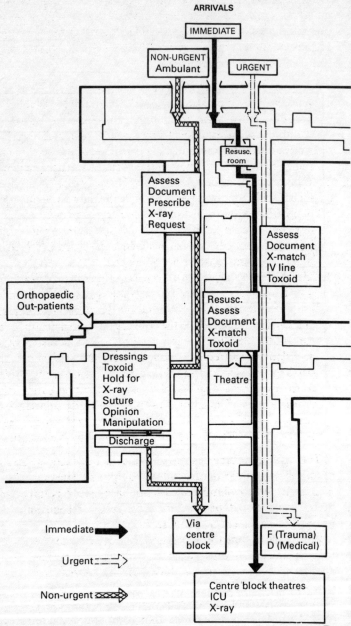

Fig. 4.2 Accident and Emergency Department major incident flow chart.

Personal knowledge of an individual's role is essential, but staff must be exercised at regular intervals if an effective state of preparation is to be achieved, and records, supplies, delegated accommodation, and equipment found suitable. Rehearsal of the plan can be at several levels.

1   Regular telephone alerting of key departments such as the A&E unit, or individual key personnel, for example, members of the hospital control team or mobile team. Alerting procedures test communication, staff availability, and time taken to respond, as well as usefully reinforcing key personnel of the need to maintain their role regarding duties in the event of a major incident.

2   Individual units or services can rehearse aspects of their own plan. Table top exercises are invaluable and have the advantage of creating minimal disturbance to normal hospital activities and have little, if any, financial implication. Ambulance and other necessary services can be involved thereby ensuring that communication and liaison roles are tested.

3   Major exercise involving all aspects of the district health authority's response, the role of the rescue services and communication are necessary from time to time but have financial implications and can have an effect on the delivery of normal health care at the time of the exercise. In view of this, such exercises are organised at relatively infrequent periods, and it is essential that all participating services should clearly understand their role prior to the exercise so that the exercise is not rendered ineffective at an early stage. Unheralded exercises utilising simulated casualties are invaluable but are best employed when the basic objectives of the plans are fully understood by participating staff.

The value of exercise is the identification of inadequacies in, for example, communication, facilities, equipment, and of aspects of the plan itself. Where simulated casualties are used it is important that their safety should be assured. This is the responsibility of the hospital management planning team.

From time to time the opportunity will arise for the health services to cooperate with other agencies who are rehearsing their own disaster plans, i.e., airports, docks, and industrial sites. This is an excellent opportunity to test communication and the coordination of plans, and does not usually mean the involvement of large numbers of staff, ambulance vehicles, or disruption of hospital services.

Conclusion

As described in this chapter, there are many different disciplines involved in handling a major incident. Communications between such groups is clearly essential, and that involves teamwork and mutual understanding. These are areas that must be addressed well in advance of any major incident, hence the need for interdisciplinary planning well in advance.

5

The mobile team
Peter Salt

A key responsibility of hospitals in the event of disaster is to provide a back up medical and nursing team able to go to the scene of the incident. In a large urban area where there is more than one major acute hospital, the responsibilities may be shared so that, for example, hospital A supplies a mobile team but hospital B accepts the majority of the casualties, with hospital A taking any overload that may occur. However, the usual pattern is for a hospital to supply a team and accept casualties.

The mobile team usually comprises a small group of personnel who are able to attend the scene of an incident at short notice, upon the request of the emergency services. Some desirable characteristics of this team are considered below.

Rapid response

The team must be available at all times and be capable of speedy dispatch whenever requested by the emergency services. Ideally, the response time should be the same as for an ambulance on a 999 call, and the team should be mobile seven minutes later.

The method of transportation varies. The majority of teams rely on a National Health Service (NHS) ambulance to take them to the scene, though some A&E units have raised funds and bought their own vehicles which have been customised to suit their needs. Such A&E units tend to be in geographically remote areas and are frequently required to send a flying squad to the scene of incidents such as road traffic accidents where casualties are trapped and in need of pain relief and resuscitation (e.g., an intravenous infusion, airway management, etc.). A flying squad is more likely to be needed if the area does not have advanced trained ambulance personnel or a local BASICS scheme (see p. 54). Another alternative means of transport is via a police vehicle, though this does impose limitations of space for transporting equipment.

One advantage of the mobile team using an NHS ambulance is that the vehicle is immediately available to transport casualties back to hospital, and the driver will have experience of high-speed emergency motoring conditions.

Personnel

The choice of personnel needs very careful consideration. Firstly, they must be readily available, thus enabling rapid mobilisation. Secondly, the personnel sent out must not denude A&E departments and other front line areas of vital staff. The third crucial point is that personnel must have the experience and knowledge to do the job expected of them in the field, i.e., rapid assessment of priorities, the initiation of emergency life-saving treatment and first aid, and the practice of triage for casualty treatment and disposal.

The aim of the mobile team is to assess and treat casualties as appropriate, to prevent deterioration, and save life. This involves the process of triage in deciding priorities for treatment on site and for removal to hospital. The team is not there to undertake long-term treatment (apart from freeing trapped casualties); its function is confined to rapid assessment, life-saving measures, and organising rapid removal to hospital for those who will benefit most from such priority.

Triage is about ensuring those most likely to benefit from immediate treatment are seen first. Professional and moral dilemmas may occur however in mass casualty situations. Priority must be given not only to those patients who have life threatening conditions but also to those who are 'salvageable'. Therefore, casualties who have such serious injuries that they will not survive even with intensive treatment have to take a lower priority. This contradicts normal practice where a severely injured casualty, whatever their injuries, is afforded maximum priority. With mass casualty over-load, this is not possible.

Taking the above discussion into account, experienced medical staff are essential for mobile team personnel. Doctors with experience in the following fields are therefore considered the most suitable.

72

1 Senior doctors with experience of managing 'polytrauma'.
2 Anaesthetists with the ability to handle resuscitation *under difficult conditions* (gaining IV access and management of the airway with endotracheal intubation are essential).
3 General surgeons proficient in making rapid and accurate diagnosis of life threatening chest and abdominal injuries. Together with head injuries, these are the most frequent causes of death in disaster situations.

The above considerations indicate that a junior casualty officer is not suitable for a mobile disaster team.

Nursing staff are also of great importance to the mobile team. Ideally, the senior nurse on the team should be drawn from the A&E unit, be of charge nurse grade, and in possession of advanced skills such as the ability to set up IVIs, thereby assisting the medical staff in this crucial task. The benefits of a senior, experienced A&E nurse heading up the nursing side of the team are obvious in that she/he will, apart from being familiar with the care of injured patients, be used to triage, rapid assessment, and decisions about priority. It is something of an A&E cliché to say, 'a little bit of blood goes a long way', but a relatively small wound can look deceptively severe to inexperienced eyes. The experienced A&E nurse will not be over-awed by such injuries.

Other nursing staff will be required to make up the team, and they too should be familiar with the care of injured patients and/or patients requiring airway management. The problem here is that the sort of nurses described are precisely the sort who are going to be needed at the hospital receiving the casualties, both in A&E, intensive care, or theatres. A careful balance has to be made between getting the right nurses to the scene, but not at the expense of reducing the effectiveness of the A&E unit or hospital generally (see Chapter 4).

Mobile team equipment

There is widespread variation in mobile team equipment in the UK, unlike countries such as Sweden and Norway where there is standardisation. If two teams are present at a major incident from different units, there are obvious advantages to standardised equipment.

The requirement of the team to be able to offer immediate life saving aid indicates the need for equipment that can be used for the ABC (airway, breathing, circulation) of resuscitation (see p. 9).

Airway protection

This requires basic equipment such as a good range of oropharyngeal airways, and advanced equipment permitting endotracheal or naso-tracheal intubation.It should be remembered that casualties may be young children, as well as adults, therefore oropharyngeal airways should range from sizes 1 to 4, and endotracheal tubes from sizes 5 to 10; cuffed and non-cuffed. Endotracheal tubes should be pre-cut to length if possible (they are usually of a generous length, which is not a problem in the controlled more leisurely atmosphere of an anaesthetic room where they can be cut exactly to size!), kept in clean packs with a good supply of lubricant, for example, KY jelly, for their introduction.

Also available should be two laryngoscopes and an endotracheal tube introducer to facilitate intubation. The laryngoscope is essential for intubation, and there should be a choice of both a straight and curved blade for each instrument, together with a paediatric blade. They must be checked regularly to ensure the light bulbs and batteries are working properly, along with the rest of the instrument, as they are literally life saving pieces of equipment.

Two 10 ml syringes for inflating the cuff, tape for tying the endotracheal tube securely in place, and non-toothed artery forceps to clamp the cuff thereby inflating the tube safely, are also needed.

A crucial piece of equipment for maintaining a clear airway is a good suction device. This must be portable and able to deliver powerful suction through either a rigid, wide bore, Yankeur-type sucker, or a long, flexible, narrow suction catheter. It is possible to obtain very effective battery driven units the size of a small briefcase, or gas cannister powered suction units. An alternative design is a hand-held, trigger/gun unit that relies on manual squeezing of the trigger to work.

Breathing

A hand-powered ventilation bag is essential to maintain breathing for a severely injured victim, e.g., Ambubag. At least three should therefore be included in the team's equipment, together with the appropriate connecting tubing to attach the bag to an oxygen supply, and catheter mounts to connect the bag to an endotracheal airway.

A major recent development is the portable, compressed oxygen powered ventilator, for example, the Oxylog or Pneupack. They automatically ventilate the patient, working simply off the pressure of the oxygen contained in an oxygen cylinder. These ventilators have now superseded the older Minuteman portable ventilators.

The treatment of pneumothorax or haemothorax (p. 33) may be a life-saving intervention on site, therefore, the appropriate intercostal drainage equipment is essential. This comprises a chest drain with trochar introducer and a one-way valve system incorporating a Heimlich flutter valve. The traditional underwater seal drainage system is not suitable for a disaster situation, hence the need to use a Heimlich valve. An improvised alternative could be the use of a catheter drainage bag such as the Simpla S4 as this is sterile and has a nonreturn valve at its neck. The introduction of a chest drain will require the use of a scalpel, injected local anaesthetic, and an aerosol skin preparation agent, while securing the drain requires the use of a straight needle and silk suture to carry out the necessary purse string closure.

The mobile team should not worry about stocking up with oxygen cylinders and masks, this equipment will be available from the ambulance service on scene.

Circulation

As described previously (p. 18), hypovolaemic shock is a major life threatening emergency and it is essential to immediately replace the fluid lost to the circulation. While blood would seem the obvious choice, there are major problems because of the need to cross match to ensure the right group is given, and blood has a short shelf life.

In the field, the intravenous (IV) fluid of choice should be a plasma expander such as Haemaccel or Gelofusine. They have a long shelf life, are easily carried and stored in 500 ml plastic containers, and have the desired properties. It should be remembered that crystalloid solutions such as normal saline or dextrose are of little value in restoring circulating volume in the polytrauma casualty.

A variety of IV cannulae are required ranging from a large, wide bore size for rapid resuscitation, to small, paediatric sizes for child and infant casualties. The Venflon design is the most commonly used. The important point however is that the IV cannulae in the mobile team equipment must be the same as that normally used in the hospital, the staff will therefore be familiar with its use. This is no place for learning new techniques! Blood infusion sets should be included with the IV fluids and, again, should include paediatric sizes as well as the usual adult variety.

Cannulae suitable for insertion into the external jugular should be included, but cannulae used for Central Venous Pressure monitoring are not needed on site. Such sophisticated techniques have their proper place in the hospital Intensive Therapy Unit (ITU).

The team's equipment should include materials for making the intravenous infusion (IVI) safe once it has been established. Fixative dressings are therefore required to prevent the cannulae dislodging and also to minimise infection risks. Splintage and bandages will assist in securing the IVI, but it should be remembered that the casualty will be subject to manhandling in a possibly difficult and hazardous environment to effect rescue and evacuation. It is unusual to find convenient objects to hang IVIs from, therefore, butchers' 'S' shaped meathooks are recommended for inclusion with the IVI equipment, together with short drip poles spiked at one end so that they can be driven into soft ground.

It may be advantageous for a casualty to have a blood specimen sent ahead to hospital for grouping and cross matching so that on arrival at hospital the appropriate blood is ready for transfusion. Needles, 20 ml syringes and specimen bottles would therefore be useful additions to the equipment. The police may be able to take samples on ahead to the hospital, subject to site security demands on their manpower. However, the danger in mass casualty situations is of misidentification, resulting in mis-matched transfusion and possibly the death of the patient. This system is therefore not practical if large numbers of casualties are involved.

As discussed previously, a major step in treating hypovolaemic shock is to stop bleeding from open wounds. This indicates the need for basic dressing packs. These dressing packs should include large surgipads and sterile irrigating solutions such as normal saline, plus antiseptic solutions, for example, povidine iodine. An irrigating solution serves a dual purpose: firstly, to wash out extensive wounds, thereby reducing contamination and facilitating assessment; and, secondly, to soak the dressing pad that is then placed over the wound. If the wound is kept moist, this will greatly assist surgical repair and healing.

Bandages are obviously essential, together with rolls of tape, safety-pins, slings and rigid cervical collars to immobilise the neck of any casualty suspected of having suffered injury to this crucial area. As the series of case studies in the second part of this book will show, there is a high probability of burns amongst the casualties. Therefore, special non-adherent burns sheets and dressings should also be included. The possibility of hypothermia, especially amongst entrapped casualties, also suggests the need for the inclusion of several foil space blankets.

This section on mobile team equipment can be concluded by considering the following basic principles which should guide planners in deciding what equipment to include in the team's packs.

1 As far as possible, it should be the same as is used in everyday hospital practice so staff are familiar with it.
2 To avoid unnecessary duplication, find out what the ambulance service carry routinely in their vehicles, but also remember to ask whether it will be enough in a disaster situation?
3 Equipment must be easily identifiable, conveniently packed, and readily accessible in the field.
4 Equipment must be portable as it may have to be manhandled through a very difficult environment, possibly in the dark, and under adverse weather conditions.
5 The function of the mobile team is triage and immediate life-saving activity; the ABC of resuscitation, *not* to set up a mobile MASH-style field hospital.

Drugs

It is important to look carefully at the drugs likely to be required in the field as there is a risk of creating an ever increasing stock to cover every possible eventuality; this is impractical.

All NHS ambulances carry Entonox gas cylinders. Entonox is 50% oxygen and 50% nitrous oxide gas and is an excellent inhalation analgesic that also has the advantage of being familiar to staff as it is widely used. It is contained in small, portable cylinders and is self-administered by the patient, which allows the patient to control their level of pain relief. The self administration characteristic of

Entonox is a useful safeguard against accidental overdose. To self administer the gas, a tight fit is essential with the mask held firmly against the face by the patient. If the patient starts to become drowsy, the mask will fall away from the face and therefore the patient will no longer be able to administer the gas. It should be remembered before undertaking a painful procedure that the gas takes some three minutes or so to have maximum effect. Its effects wear off just as quickly when the patient stops breathing the gas, therefore continual administration is essential for effective pain relief.

For moderate to severe pain, the current drug of choice is Nalbuphine Hydrochloride (Nubain). This has the advantage of not depressing respiration or leading to a diminished level of consciousness, both of which are side effects of potent narcotic drugs such as morphine. It may be given by injection, via the intravenous, intramuscular or subcutaneous route, in a dose of 10–20 mg for the average 70 kg (154 lb) adult.

For the control of severe pain, the practical means still remains the traditional narcotic or opiate group of drugs such as morphine or papaveretum (Omnopon). However, there are side effects, as mentioned above. It is not possible to give a head injured patient narcotic analgesia, as any subsequent deterioration in consciousness, which is a cardinal sign of brain related injury and therefore an indication for urgent neurosurgical management, could be simply due to the drug. Vital signs may therefore be masked by the side effects of the narcotic analgesic drug in the head injured casualty. The depressant effect on respiration is another unwanted side effect. Narcotic drugs are also subject to the Controlled Drug Act which imposes strict regulations on their storage and usage.

Other useful drugs may be listed as follows:

diuretics, e.g., frusemide
corticosteroids, e.g., Solu-Medrone
heparinised saline to keep IV cannulae patent if no drip is being run.
antiemetics, e.g., Metoclopromide. Another side effect of narcotics is to induce nausea.
A short acting anaesthetic such as Ketalar as a surgical procedure may be necessary to free a trapped victim, for example, amputation of a limb.
Muscle relaxants to facilitate intubation. These should be stored in a

fridge as they need to be kept at a constant low temperature. The take out drug packs should be clearly labelled with the whereabouts of muscle relaxant drugs to ensure they are not forgotten.

Standard packs of cardiac arrest drugs; it has to be said that a patient suffering cardiac arrest on site would either have been resuscitated by an ambulance crew before the mobile team arrived, or, in a mass casualty situation, have been abandoned as beyond help, such is the nature of triage in these situations. A patient may suffer cardiac arrest after the team arrives, but in these situations it is difficult to know how much time the team will have available for treatment as the patient would be placed in a low survival expectancy category.

In discussing drugs it can be seen that it is essential the variety is kept to the bare minimum, i.e., the drugs which are required to aid the function of a mobile team. A good supply of needles and syringes is essential for drug administration and, in addition, staff must be very careful in checking that the correct doses are given and the type, quantity, and amount of drug given must be recorded for each patient. This is essential information for the hospital medical staff. Simple methods of recording drug administration include writing with an indelible marker on the casualty's body; a more sophisticated method is discussed later (p. 81).

Packaging of equipment

Packs to carry the equipment should be readily portable, and as light as possible, but also robust and waterproof. They should be clearly marked and worded as hospital mobile equipment, including the name and logo of the hospital base. The scene of a disaster can be a very chaotic place and it would be very easy for hospital packs to go missing or become mixed up with the equipment of the other services such as the fire brigade. Packs should include shoulder straps to facilitate carrying and be of a bright colour.

Many containers are in use for carrying drugs, but the best in my experience is a steel tool-box of concertina shelf design. It allows plenty of room and the contents can all be easily seen as it is opened out. Handles for carrying and the ability to lock the box securely with a padlock are great advantages, together with the protection it affords to the fragile glass ampoules within. The box should be a bright colour and clearly marked as hospital property, though the word 'drugs' should be omitted for security reasons.

Protective clothing

The clothing required will have to be adaptable to a wide range of situations. Kitting out a full team is a very expensive business and therefore mistakes in clothing are going to be expensive mistakes, mistakes that should not occur with correct planning and discussion.

The requirements of clothing are; that it should protect staff from injury due to hazards on scene, the weather (cold and wet), and make them readily visible and identifiable for their own protection. The traditional hospital uniforms of white coats over normal day clothes for doctors and nurses uniforms are totally unsuitable for a disaster scene, even if it is a fine summer's day.

The account of the Tottenham Riots on p. 140 gives further points for consideration. A team working on site for several hours will soon cease to function effectively if they become wet and cold. Conversely, as the account of the IRA bombing campaign in London on p. 131 shows, the mobile team may have to work in sweltering heat on a midsummer's afternoon. The following apparel has been tried and tested and is therefore recommended, but it should be available in a wide range of sizes to reflect the diversity of the human frame. This means that eight sets of clothing and footwear may be needed to be sure of equipping a team of four.

Thermal 'all in one' jumpsuits. These comprise trousers and top all in one garment and, with ordinary underwear underneath, are very effective.

Boilersuits. These are good robust garments with plenty of useful pockets. They allow easy mobility and, covering the whole body, afford substantial protection. They may be readily worn in conjunction with one of the jumpsuits mentioned above.

Full weatherproof suits of the oilskin type, or at least trousers of this material, are essential for working in foul weather conditions or where there is a risk of chemical spillage. Apart from the protection they afford, they can make it easy for staff to be decontaminated by the fire brigade.

Fluorescent jackets. These should be loose fitting and have plenty of pockets. They also make the wearer readily visible.

All the above items should be clearly marked to indicate that the wearer is a member of the hospital medical team to avoid confusion on scene. Many staff from the other services will also be wearing fluorescent jackets and tabards, so easy identification is vital to avoid confusion.

Footwear. Ordinary duty shoes are of no value in a disaster situation. Staff must be equipped with *chemical resistant* wellington boots with thermal inners and/or socks.

Gloves. Heavy-duty gloves are essential. Woollen mittens are also useful to allow more delicate tasks to be carried out.

Helmets. Ideally they should be of a miner's design that can be fitted with a battery powered headlight and should have a secure fastening strap. A helmet is of no value if it falls off the first time the wearer moves his/her head. The helmet should also carry a medical team logo or at least a prominent red cross for identification purposes.

Other personal equipment. Heavy-duty, plastic handled scissors are invaluable for a variety of tasks such as the removal of clothing. A hand torch should be carried with a protective rubber casing and ring for attachment to clothing. Indellible markers, pens and pencils are essential, together with identity triage cards, see below.

Identity triage cards

During the first phase of triage on scene, the use of a colour coded triage card is most useful. The card opens out into a cross shape with each arm of the cross a different colour according to the following criteria:

red   = priority
yellow = can wait
green = must wait
black = dead

Once a decision has been made about priority, the card is folded in such a way that the appropriate colour is shown. A body outline on the reverse side may then be marked to show injuries and a note made of any medication given, plus any other relevant information. The card is then placed in a transparent, protective, plastic wallet and secured around the patient's neck. The information contained about the patient's condition on leaving the scene will be invaluable for the A&E staff performing second level triage at the hospital. This method is a more sophisticated variation of the military system where the actual body is marked, for example, with an 'M' on the forehead indicating morphine has been given.

In Chapter 10 there is an account of the Tottenham riots, a major civil disturbance. If hospital teams are ever required to attend such incidents, the possibility of confusion with police officers in riot equipment must be considered. If such a situation were to occur, the lives of hospital staff would be at risk, as they would be considered 'legitimate' targets by the rioters. The ambulance service are at great pains to identify themselves as separate from the police for precisely this reason. Ambulance crews are issued with white helmets and clearly marked fluorescent tunics and tabards displaying a prominent red cross. Flame retardent clothing, helmets with visors, and neck guards should be available to any hospital staff required to go into a riot situation, together with clear identification. The mobile team's safety depends upon such precautions.

In concluding this section it must be stressed that all equipment and clothing should be checked regularly and thoroughly. The team will depend upon this equipment at the scene, and, if something is missing or not working, there will be no alternative source of supply.

Staff must be confident about their roles and know what they are doing. It is important for them to remember not only what they have got available, but also what is *not* available to them in the field. The field situation is nothing like the well lit, warm, controlled environment of a hospital!

Control and action on site

On arrival at the scene, the mobile team must initially make contact with the site controller. This will usually be the senior police officer present, as the police have overall responsibility for site security. At this stage, the team should ask for and receive a briefing on the situation before the controller then directs them to an area set aside for their use.

The team need to set up a casualty collecting point (CCP) in this area. Key points are that the location should be adjacent to the incident site, but also safe. Good access is essential both for bringing casualties from the immediate disaster scene, and for ambulances to evacuate casualties to hospital.

Extrication of casualties from the wreckage is the responsibility of the emergency services, especially the fire brigade. The medical team should therefore stay at the CCP where they are needed. The scene of a disaster is potentially a very dangerous area, especially for persons lacking the experience of the fire brigade and other services. Live electrical wires, leaking fuel and unstable masonry are just three possible hazards, while, in a bombing, staff should remember that a common IRA/Irish National Liberation Army (INLA) tactic is to plant more than one bomb, or other devices used to disrupt rescue work, if not aimed directly at members of the rescue and security services.

It may, however, be necessary for staff to go into the immediate disaster area to provide emergency care for trapped victims or to certify death before body removal. In such circumstances, they should always be accompanied by members of the emergency services and act under their guidance. The hazardous nature of disaster sites cannot be overemphasised.

Triage and emergency treatment should otherwise be carried out at the CCP with the medical team waiting for patients to be brought to them. One further advantage of this system is that if the other services want a doctor and nurse immediately, they know where to find them, and do not have to go roaming over the scene, possibly in poor lighting conditions, looking for urgently needed staff.

Special local factors

In addition to the general incident that can happen anywhere such as a train crash, A&E units need to think about special local circumstances and the implication this has for planning and equipment. For example, the presence of a large chemical or nuclear plant poses unique hazards. It may be possible that the hospital team have to work in respirators, for example, and the hospital plan has to consider widespread environmental contamination from toxic chemicals or radioactive material. Likewise, in a mining area, it is possible that the team will have to work underground.

If the A&E unit is situated in a coastal area close to major shipping routes, especially if a busy ferry port is involved, the planning will need to allow for the possibility of a maritime incident. The hospital team may be required to operate offshore, and therefore close liaison with the coastguard, Royal National Lifeboat Institution (RNLI), or the Royal Navy at the planning stage is required in addition to the usual services.

Action cards

Reference has already been made in Chapter 4 to the importance of action cards for individual staff members as an *aide-mémoire* to key functions. It goes without saying that such cards are essential for both the medical and nursing members of the hospital mobile team.

Rehearsal and practice

The most carefully designed plan and well-equipped mobile team are of no avail if the individual staff members are unaware of their roles. This raises the question of rehearsal and practice. This may be achieved in several ways, beginning with the standby situation, which is a desirable feature of any hospital plan.

Standby should take place when there is an incident requiring the emergency services to deploy their resources in advance of a possible major event. Examples might be an aeroplane that has informed the airport it is having difficulty with its landing equipment or is making an emergency landing for some other reason, or a major hostage incident.

For this to occur, the emergency services must notify the hospital that they are going to standby themselves and deploy their own resources accordingly. Nothing is more galling for A&E staff than to find out via the grapevine that there is a standby situation because of an aeroplane in difficulty, but they have not been officially told.

The standby facility gives the hospital service time to consider how its existing resources may need to be redeployed and also allows a period of preparation. This is desirable, rather than having to activate the procedure immediately. In the worst situations, the only notification the hospital has is the arrival of mass casualties.

The various steps that are taken during a standby phase offer an excellent training opportunity. It should never be looked upon as overdramatising the situation or a false alarm. How easy was it to contact certain personnel? How long did it take to clear the department of patients? How long did the mobile team take to get assembled and changed into appropriate clothing? Questions such as these and an analysis of unforeseen problems that occurred are essential steps in improving the plan, while the standby exercise itself would have been valuable practice and as such must be taken seriously with a proper debrief afterwards.

A formal exercise in the field may be thought of as the ideal solution, but such events take a great deal of organising, cost money that is in scarce supply, and lead to disruption of day-to-day services. A further problem is getting staff to take them seriously. If staff regard the exercise as a bit of a joke and fail to take it seriously, it will be of little value.

The disruption involved in the main A&E unit may be limited to some extent by rehearsing the mobile team's role only. Exercises called by HM Inspector of Fires, for example, provide an excellent opportunity to test out the hospital team's effectiveness. Alternative scenarios may occur locally when, say, a major building is to be demolished, giving the team experience of getting to an urban location quickly and working in an environment closely resembling the chaotic aftermath of a bombing or building collapse. The medical branches of the armed services hold regular exercises and there may be value in hospitals establishing links with, for example, territorial reserve units to explore any ways in which such military exercises may benefit hospital staff.

Conclusion

The hospital medical team can offer a vital, life-saving treatment and triage service on site. To do this, however, the medical team needs to be able to get on scene as soon as possible after the incident has occurred. The team should consist of staff with the right experience and knowledge, who are properly equipped and prepared, and in possession of a clear plan of action.

Does your hospital team meet those criteria?

6

The role of the local authority emergency planning officer

Most people are familiar with the roles of the various emergency services such as the police force and fire brigade. However, the functioning of the Emergency Planning Officer (EPO) and his team tends to remain less well-known. Although very much in the background and not involving the high profile on site of the other emergency services, the EPO team have a crucial role to play in major incidents, an area that will be explored in this short chapter.

Emergency planning teams were established in 1972, following the disbandment of the Civil Defence Corps in 1968, and operate under general Home Office guidelines. Their brief was to plan and to coordinate local authority services in the event of a major peacetime disaster or other similar emergency, in addition to continuing to have responsibility for civil defence planning in the event of war. It is the peacetime emergency part of their role that will be discussed here. In the UK, at present, there are 69 county or equivalent EPOs together with supporting staff.

EPOs have approached their planning problems from the point of view of having a general plan to cover a major emergency anywhere in their area, e.g., the evacuation and temporary shelter of a section of the population. They have then gone on to look at specific high-risk sites within their area to try and anticipate and plan for contingencies that may arise. This ranges from man-made accidents involving major chemical plants and nuclear power stations on the one hand, through to natural disasters such as extensive flooding, marine or riverine in origin.

Their role has become more important than ever after the introduction of the Control of Industrial Major Accident Hazards Regulations (CIMAH) in 1984. These regulations list over 300 different toxic agents and set limits, and any plant holding such agents in excess of the set limit must have both an on site and off site plan to deal with emergencies. The health and safety executive and also the implementation of planning permission regulations will alert the authorities to the need to apply CIMAH regulations to any plant. The company then have six months to provide on site plans. At the same time, an off site plan has to be prepared by the local authority, a matter normally coordinated by the EPO team acting in liaison with the company and all the relevant emergency services. If they have not already done so, hospital major disaster planning teams should familiarise themselves with any such installations within their catchment area and the nature of plans that have been drawn up.

The county or equivalent team operates a 24 hour on-call system. The basic function of the team is to mobilise local authority or other resources which are needed by the emergency services in the field. They are therefore normally removed from the scene of the incident, but form a crucial communication channel through which many different services may coordinate their operations. However, in some cases and in some specific plans, the EPO may deploy staff members to the site of operations where they would be in direct communication with headquarters (HQ).

It is essential that EPO HQ has good communications with local town halls if they are to coordinate resources effectively. A typical set up involves both direct land lines bypassing the telephone system, and also radio communication, giving EPO HQ two different modes of communication with local town halls. If a teleprinter is included in this system, then direct transmission of hard copy is possible, greatly facilitating speedy communication. A recent advance has involved the installation of a new keyboard and visual display unit (VDU) system, operated via landline, for civil defence purposes. This links the county or equivalent HQ direct with emergency centres and also with the police and Home Office officials. This system is intended for civil defence, but the Civil Protection in Peacetime Act of 1986 authorises its use in a peacetime emergency. It is possible therefore for an EPO HQ to have three separate and secure modes of communication with the local town hall emergency room or centre, a great advantage in the event of a major incident.

In addition to having direct communications with local authorities, the EPO HQ also links up to the police, fire brigade, ambulance service and armed services, and many HQs are also installing direct links with their Regional Health Authority. These are usually radio links.

The resources that the EPO team can make available in the field are described below. For example, within a shire county the County Surveyor's Department has great resources of manpower and equipment (earthmoving plants, etc.) together with expert knowledge in fields such as roads and buildings. The department will also know where to obtain extra equipment from the private sector to supplement local authority resources. Liaison with the public utilities, for example, gas, water and electricity is greatly facilitated by the surveyor's department as they are used to working with such services on a routine basis.

The other major resources that the EPO team will be able to mobilise are based in social services and education departments. The former will be able to provide rest centres and personnel with invaluable experience in dealing with social emergencies, essential in any relocation exercise, together with supplies of emergency clothing and bedding either from their own resources or through liaison with voluntary organisations such as the WRVS or Salvation Army. The education department are also able to provide temporary shelter in schools. Schools are well-suited to this purpose as the playground provides vehicular access and car parking space, there are toilet and usually cooking facilities within, and the buildings are spacious and well heated. In some counties, however, the education department's primary role is that of providing nourishment to evacuees.

Other resources may be called upon as required, for example, the county analyst to provide scientific analysis of an incident. Many counties and districts are now, in the post-Chernobyl era, looking into setting up their own radiation monitoring schemes to provide a rapid and independent service. One such lead in this has been given by Lancashire County Council together with the 14 District Councils in Lancashire who have set up their own scheme (Radiation Monitoring in Lancashire – RADMIL). The Lancashire scheme was set up before Chernobyl and therefore allowed the EPO to monitor the effects on the county accurately, especially as there was a good baseline of data prior to the incident for comparison.

Most local authorities are required to activate their EPO teams several times per year. Their function is therefore far from a paper and planning exercise. Consider, as a typical example, the county of

Lancashire, located between the high and very wet Pennines to the east, and a low lying coast to the west facing the Irish Sea which is prone to tidal storm surges in the same way as the North Sea. Not surprisingly, major inundations due to either tidal or riverine flooding do happen involving the mobilisation of the emergency services over a wide area.

Lancashire is very well-known as an industrial county and there are substantial quantities of potentially very dangerous chemicals located in various factories and moving on the roads and railways of the area. The nuclear industry is present with the Heysham A and Heysham B Nuclear Power Stations, a major British Nuclear Fuels Limited (BNFL) plant at Springfields, and also many of the spent nuclear fuel flasks en route to BNFL Sellafield in Cumbria, next door to Lancashire across Morecambe Bay, travel the length of the county on the busy west coast main railway line. One of the busiest stretches of motorway in the country, M6/M61/M56, crosses the county in both north–south and east–west directions, small wonder there have been major accidents with many deaths. See p. 181 for an account of one such incident.

As if this is not enough, the county boasts the popular resort of Blackpool, popular with major political parties as a conference venue, in addition to the day-trippers out for a day beside the sea. In view of the IRA bombing at Brighton, which came very close to assassinating the Prime Minister, party conferences provide another major planning headache. The major security operations surrounding the Conservative Party's return to Brighton for their annual conference in 1988 confirms the seriousness of the problem.

These are just a few of the areas that the county EPO team are fully involved with, in addition to radiation monitoring. Yet it is doubtful if even they could have anticipated a water authority pumping station exploding as a party of local villagers were being shown round, but this is, of course, exactly what happened at Abbeystead (see p. 172). In this situation, the EPO team were called out to mobilise county council resources. They also arranged for refreshments to be provided for the 150 or so emergency personnel who worked long into the night amongst the underground rubble of the pumping station. A small point perhaps, but if rescue personnel are not able to get a sandwich and a cup of tea when they need it, it must start to reduce the level at which they are functioning. In this instance, tea was provided into the small hours of the morning via a Salvation Army mobile kitchen based in Blackburn and staff from Preston, care of the EPO team!

Conclusion

The function of the EPO HQ can be summarised as follows:

1   It provides an essential planning and coordinating function for a major incident involving a wide range of services.
2   It permits speedy and secure communication with local authorities, the emergency services, armed forces and government agencies, bypassing the inevitable log jam of ordinary telephone lines.
3   It can make available to the emergency services a wide range of resources, manpower and expertise.
4   It permits evacuation and relocation of the population.
5   In the event of an incident of major proportions with national implications, the EPO HQ is a vital link in the chain necessary to mobilise national resources, via government.
6   The existence of a professional full-time cadre of emergency planners allows for a sharing of experience and knowledge across the country. This is a point that will be returned to in the final chapter of the book.

7

The psychology of disaster
Mary N. Haslum

Disasters are frequently described in quantitative and statistical terms: the number of dead and injured, the extent of damage to buildings and other physical resources, the number of homeless, the ultimate economic costs. Yet for both victims and helpers it is the suffering the disaster brings – the human terror, anguish and despair that is most vital. . . . The experiences of a disaster and the emotions felt are remembered and relived, and are not readily extinguished in either the vividness of their imagery or the reliving of the emotions. Anguish at death, destruction, and the loss of loved ones, the destruction of home and place may give way to despair when the victims realise that, although they have survived and must continue to do so, life can never be the same again.

(Raphael, 1986: p. 29)

Four terrible disasters passed into history in Britain in 1987. These were the capsize of a roll-on/roll-off ferry, *The Herald of Free Enterprise*, at Zeebrugge in Belgium, the Hungerford shootings, the Enneskillen bombing and the fire in King's Cross St Pancras underground station. Other disasters are described in the later chapters of this book. One of the developments from disasters such as these has been the growing realisation that people caught up in these situations may suffer not only physical damage but also considerable psychological damage. Clegg (1988) has commented that, while in this country the life-saving services have debriefings as a matter of routine, the concept of psychological debriefings is virtually unknown. Consequently, understanding of the psychological problems, which people caught up in these situations have to overcome, is far from complete.

Temporal dimensions of a disaster

It is now being realised that rather than being short-lived events, disasters have long time-spans as far as the people caught up in them are concerned. The period of disaster begins with a *warning* phase in which it is often possible to recognise that conditions are present which could lead to a disaster. This is followed by a phase of *threat* when there are specific indicators of an approaching disaster. The *impact* stage covers the period of injury, death and destruction: the fire is actually raging, the earth convulsing or the shots being fired. This is followed by an *inventory* stage when those exposed to the disaster take stock of what has happened to them and this overlaps with the *rescue* stage when the injured are helped either by people who have not been hurt or by those who have come to help. The *remedy* stage covers the period where specific formal steps are taken to bring relief to affected people. *Recovery* is the very long subsequent period in which individuals adjust to their altered personal circumstances: learning to live without loved ones, new surroundings and social groups, coping with disability, or maybe adapting to different employment. It will certainly include coming to terms with the experience of the disaster.

This model of disaster, suggested by Powell (1954), can be summarised as:

pre-disaster-warning – threat – impact – inventory – rescue – remedy – recovery conditions

It provides a framework for thinking about the behaviour, emotional experiences and psychological suffering of people caught up in disaster and emergency situations.

Spatial dimensions of a disaster

There are several categories of affected people whom it is useful to identify beyond the obvious category of victim and rescuer. To understand these it is helpful to realise that disasters occur not only in time but also in space. The area of *primary impact* is surrounded by an area of *partial impact* which is surrounded by the *outside community* (Wallace, 1975). Destruction, death and disruption vary with distance from the area of primary impact.

Victims

Whilst the obvious victims are found in the primary impact area and are those who have been directly affected or hurt, other people may not have been in or near the primary impact area at the time of the disaster but nevertheless been terribly affected through loss of loved ones, property or sources of livelihood. Often, the first rescuers are in the primary impact area. Victims help other victims and so assume dual roles of victim and rescuer. The next rescuers on the scene may come from the partial impact zone and take on the role of rescuer, whilst themselves not being unaffected by the impact. Later, rescuers come from the unaffected outside community.

Although there may be a merging of victim and rescuer roles, Short (1979) has warned that the stereotypes attached to these two roles can prevent this from being recognised. Victims are helpless, vulnerable and weak. Rescuers are helpful, invulnerable and strong. Where victims are recognised as rescuers they may be labelled heroes, but it may not always be realised that a rescuer has also been a victim, nor that a rescuer can become a victim. Kliman (1976) called such people, 'the hidden victims of the disaster'.

Taylor and Frazer (1981) suggested six categories of victims: primary victims were people in the impact area who received maximum exposure; secondary victims were the grieving relatives and friends; third level victims were rescue and recovery workers who needed help and support to keep going and might need help later to adjust to what they were going through; fourth level victims were people in the community (non-trained helpers or those who shared in the grief and loss); fifth level victims were not directly involved but became very distressed by the disaster; and sixth level victims were not involved in the disaster but might have been primary victims if some element of chance had not prevented it.

Apart from the victim role of being weak and resourceless, they are often expected to be grateful for rescue and help. How do you express your grief, anger and distress as you need if the people helping you keep expecting you to be grateful? Special relationships do develop between victims and their helpers but some of these may only work as long as the helper feels they are helping or needed, and in control.

93

Helpers

A helper also has many role expectations. They are expected to know what is going on, to be able to act, to be in control, to succeed. Helpers help for many different reasons and each brings her/his own experiences, ideas and reasons for helping into the situation. She/he may be a trained member of the emergency care services, either professional or volunteer. What she/he is required to do in an emergency situation may be similar to everyday experience or very different. The role adopted can be affected by how clearly the immediate goals of the situation and the lines of command are defined. Some helpers will be untrained, and will never have faced such a situation before, but are in the impact area and able and willing to help.

Bystanders

Some people come to watch and stay to help whilst many come only to watch. Bystanders come from the partial impact area or the outside community. In some situations bystanders can cause the rescue services real problems in making access to disaster areas difficult. In one sense at least, the media defining disasters as 'news' turns anyone with a television or a newspaper into a bystander.

Several domains of psychological enquiry provide clues as to what goes on in disaster and emergency situations, and some have been selected for discussion here within the context of the disaster stages outlined. The areas considered include accident research, information processing and decision making from cognitive psychology, the psychophysiology of stress, social psychological approaches to bystander intervention, and the psychology of loss and bereavement.

Most of this book is concerned with disaster management. The action and interaction of groups of health care workers is considered alongside the procedures they follow in different disaster and emergency situations. In this chapter an attempt is made to focus on individuals caught up in disasters, and to ask questions such as: 'What makes an individual vulnerable?'; 'What makes her/him refuse to heed warnings?'; 'How can a disaster affect someone caught up in it?'; 'How can models of stress help us understand how to help victims and rescuers?'; 'Can you get over a disaster?'; 'What influences bystander intervention?'; 'What kinds of psychological aftercare may victims and helpers need?'.

Psychological factors in disaster situations form a huge topic and this discussion can in no way be comprehensive; rather it is the intention to pull together some disparate areas of psychological enquiry and to examine their relevance to the experiences of individuals caught up in disaster and emergency situations. An excellent text for a comprehensive and sensitive examination of the issues is provided by Raphael (1986); some of her ideas are presented in the discussion which follows.

Psychological factors in pre-disaster conditions

It is tempting to view disasters as stemming either from human error or natural hazards, but there are an increasing number of disaster and emergency situations where the causal factors are deliberate and premeditated actions intended to maim and destroy human life.

Accidents on a large scale, particularly those which involve injury to people, assume the mantle of disasters. Arbous and Kerrich (1951) defined an accident as, 'an unplanned event in a chain of planned and controlled events'. It is worthwhile, therefore, to consider briefly some of the psychological factors in the antecedents of accidents.

Accident proneness

One of the most controversial topics in accident research has been whether some people are more prone to accidents than others. Is accident proneness a permanent state of an individual or does it fluctuate with changing conditions and experience?

Most people tend to avoid situations where they may get hurt and take extra care in the presence of real danger and yet some individuals appear to lurch from one traumatic episode to another.

In accidents the results of certain actions may be visible but never the actions themselves. In addition, we rarely have records of behaviour which might, or should have, caused an accident but did not, e.g., sailing from harbour with the ferry doors not properly closed. To this extent it is possible to make erroneous inferences about an individual's liability or proneness to have an accident and consequently there is no clear-cut answer to the question.

The psychology of disaster

Personal invulnerability

Few of us spend time thinking about the disasters which may happen to us. We live in a potentially dangerous world, but if we were constantly fearful and watching for something to happen, we should do little else. Many individuals not only do not think about the possibility of a disaster, but will act, even under conditions of great risk, as though the disaster could not possibly happen to them. Look at the speeds at which people drive in poor weather conditions on motorways for evidence of this. It is not only motorists, swimmers ignore danger flags, climbers go out on mountains in poor weather conditions and so on. We appear to carry with us a sense of personal invulnerability, a belief that we ourselves cannot be involved in an accident or caught up in a disaster.

Risk assessment

When we do contemplate the possibility of an accident or disaster we weigh up the nature of the threat and the various risks. This involves asking questions like: 'How many times has it happened before?'; 'What would happen to me?'; 'What are the likely effects on others?'; 'What are the possible effects on the place where I live?'; 'How severe might these effects be?'.

An important question related to risk assessment concerns the consequences that follow the recognition of the risk. If nothing can be done, or we believe nothing can be done, a serious risk assessment may not even be made (Raphael, 1986). Why worry about it, you cannot do anything about it if it does happen? Institutions and communities, as well as individuals, all need to make risk assessments. How was it that so many people were prepared to live within the shadow of the spoil heaps at Aberfan? How will the Piper Alpha disaster affect the workforce on oil rigs? Many people live in villages by rivers which burst their banks and overwhelm flood prevention schemes. Similarly, in Australia, semirural areas of bush and dry foliage provide a delightful natural environment in which to live, but it is one which carries with it a very high risk of fire. It appears that in the cost benefit analysis of living in a particular environment, assessments of risks of potential disaster are counterbalanced by aesthetic, personal and economic factors such as, 'It is a lovely place to live'; 'Such a friendly village'; 'All my family is here'; 'We could not afford to move'.

Raphael (1986) argues that few communities have readily accessible public information on the likelihood and relative risks of natural hazards. People are rarely aware of what may happen to them and how. When risk assessments are made, they tend not to be accurate, and it is not surprising that people are sometimes poorly prepared to collaborate with authorities in preparing for a disaster.

In addition, collaboration with authorities involves tricky issues like obeying instructions or giving up personal freedoms for the safety of others, e.g., not lighting fires for a picnic on a dry moor, staying within speed limits or keeping away from dangerous areas.

Limited information processing

When a human operator is carrying out a skill such as monitoring a radar screen in an air traffic control room, checking readings in a power station control room or driving a train, she/he is processing a great deal of information. She/he is receiving signals and responding to them, forming a link between incoming information and outgoing responses.

A significant advance in understanding information processing came with the work of Miller, Gallanter and Pribram (1960) who proposed a cybernetic unit in human cognition which they called a TOTE. This stands for Test–Operate–Test–Exit. Such a model suggests that a key element in human information processing is feedback, and that information processing is a self-regulatory process of planning and checking. We can alter the sequence of mental operations in the light of feedback. However, the process can fail.

Current information processing theories further suggest that sometimes we carry out several mental operations simultaneously. A distinction can be made between two types of information processing: *controlled* and *automatic* (Hunt and Lansman, 1986; Kahneman and Treisman, 1984). Controlled operations such as repairing a watch or writing a report require conscious attention and are so highly demanding of processing resources that they have to proceed serially, one at a time. Automatic processing, on the other hand, uses minimal processing resources and many operations can be carried out in parallel, i.e., without conscious attention. Think of all the things we do driving a car, and we may listen to the radio as well.

Many accidents occur in situations which require controlled processing. Automatic processing resources are being used to the full and individuals find themselves with too much information to process in too little time. This sort of problem may occur in an emergency at a nuclear power plant, for example, see Chapter 15.

In situations like avoiding a falling object, slipping on a pavement, avoiding an obstruction, we have to switch from our highly organised automatic information processing system to the slower controlled processing mode. Kay (1971) suggested that it was at the point of changeover from one system to the other that an individual became the most vulnerable. Motorway disasters can be considered in this light, for example.

Response stereotypy

It is always difficult to assess how far an accident can be attributed to the design of equipment, but an operator, perhaps under stress, could make a wrong response because the direction of control was incompatible with the intended action. If designing a vertical lever to alter pressure in a boiler, should the bottom position of the lever be zero or maximum? If it was horizontal, should the zero be at the left or the right? Our tendency to always do things in one particular way is called response stereotypy. Remember the last time you changed your car and found the windscreen wiper and traffic indicator levers were on the 'wrong' sides. How often did you wipe the windows before turning a corner, and, if you sometimes get bothered driving do you ever repeat that mistake?

Fatigue

Much psychological research has been carried out on how performance varies with time on the job and as external conditions change, such as temperature, humidity and noise. Hebb (1955) suggested that there is an optimal level of arousal for an optimal level of performance. If arousal increases or decreases too much from this level, performance deteriorates.

Studies with vigilance tasks have shown that human operators perform badly when tired. Physical fatigue has comparatively little effect on vigilance performance, whilst mental fatigue brings about considerable deterioration (Fraser, 1958). Clearly if the demands of the situation remain the same but our ability to process the information and respond decreases, the probability of an information processing error increases. In reading the accounts of disaster and emergency situations later in this book, notice how often human error can be identified as 'a' and sometimes 'the' most likely causal factor.

Psychological factors in the warning and threat stages of a disaster

Individuals' decision making

When placed in a situation where we interpret information as indicating that an emergency situation is imminent, we are faced with a number of decisions about our actions. Janis and Mann (1977) proposed a model of the decision processes which had to be worked through in response to an authentic warning of impending danger. It was made up of questions such as:

Are the risks serious if no protective action is taken?
  If 'no', action is not necessary and no conflict is present;
  If 'maybe' or 'yes':
Are the risks serious even if action is taken?
  If 'no', action is not necessary and no conflict is present;
  If 'maybe' or 'yes':
Is there a better hope of means of escape?
  If 'no', take defensive avoidance;
  If 'maybe' or 'yes':
Is there time to do this?
  If 'no', action may may be hypervigilance or possibly panic;
  If 'maybe' or 'yes' action will be vigilance and appropriate coping
    behaviour.

This is essentially a TOTE model where feedback on decisions and consequent responses provide further information for the next decision.

Individuals, however, respond to warnings in different ways even when the warning message is clear and constant. We can hear and perceive the same message differently depending on who we are, where we are and who we are with.

Recent disaster experience and proximity to the potential disaster increase the likelihood of responding quickly and appropriately to warnings. It is worth remembering that people in the emergency services are much more likely to have had these experiences before than the people caught up in the disaster or emergency situation.

Preparedness

In 1980, Mount St Helens' volcano in South Washington State, USA, erupted. This volcano had not erupted since 1857 and consequently few people expected it to erupt. Early in 1980, the volcano started to emit steam and there were small eruptions of ash and debris. Its interest lies in the example it provided of how a population can be prepared for a major disaster effectively. Perry and Greene (1982) investigated the degree to which hazard awareness influenced the extent to which people prepared for the emergency of the volcano erupting. The study was possible because of the long lead-in time of over a month to the emergency.

Most people developed a general plan of what they would do. Those in the Primary Impact Area made specific plans which included evacuation of home and family. County sheriff's offices acted as key points in a communication network where information and specific advice was available to individual enquirers. The mass media, and television in particular, played an important role in increasing general awareness of the risk of eruption and constantly updating the public with information on which to make risk assessments. Being prepared for a situation, however, also depends on the believing the warning. It appeared that contact with the county sheriff's offices served to encourage warning belief (see Chapter 8).

Content of the warning was all-important. The more specific it was, the more likely people were to make plans and take specific actions. The whole experience showed, that given enough time to develop an appropriate communications network, it was possible to raise the level of preparedness in the population sufficiently to minimise the effects of the impact when the volcano eventually erupted.

Failing or refusing to respond to warning

Not everyone, however, responds to warning. Belief in personal invulnerability, coupled with a belief that lightning cannot strike in the same place twice, can make some people very difficult to warn.

Studies of floods and forest fires suggest that with age there may be a differential responsiveness to warnings. Elderly people are often pictured as more unwilling to be evacuated. Experience of previous disasters may have increased their personal invulnerability rather than made them 'disaster-wise', or they may be unwilling to face all the upheaval of evacuation. They may be less concerned about the possibility of their own survival and more willing to risk the consequences of inaction.

Disasters without warnings

Some disasters such as explosions, air crashes, even earthquakes can occur without warning. Stanley (1988) describing her experience of an earthquake in New Zealand says:

> In the early afternoon, people in the Whakatane area and far beyond heard loud, deep rumblings culminating in a terrific crunch. A huge chasm ripped a path of destruction across farms, forests and roads as it made its way inland from an epicentre out at sea. We felt a rapid succession of earthquakes, the largest of which measured 6.3 on the Richter scale, and their shallowness made them more devastating. The ground rolled like the sea and in the worst places it rose over three feet high. The effect was immediate as factories rocked, storage tanks collapsed, power pylons crumpled, railway lines buckled and snapped and all the mains electricity cut out. Everything stopped . . .
>
> (Stanley, 1988: p. 143)

In such situations, the shock and disorientation which people experience can be very great.

Psychological factors in the impact and inventory stages

Shock

In disasters without warning the shock which people experience can be very great and have long lasting consequences. The people who experienced the first atomic bomb in Hiroshima did not expect it, did not know what had happened, did not know what to believe. The timing added to the sense of unreality as people were just getting up and going to work. In fact, the time at which a disaster occurs appears to have a role in the extent of the shock experienced.

We expect to be safe at night when we sleep. Being woken rudely in the middle of the night finds us in an extremely vulnerable position any way – being woken by an explosion in the night, as in the recent bombing of the Mill Hill Barracks in London, must have been a particularly frightening and disorienting experience.

The physical and sensory elements of the impact are not within usual experience (see Stanley, 1988, in the previous section). For most of us the intensity of the environmental changes; the blast of sound and air, the heat of the fire, the smell of the dust and debris are outside our experience and beyond our imagination.

In severe shock, an individual may feel her/himself to be in a trance-like state, detached from ordinary reality, even from her or his own body and may feel no pain. McDermott (1980) suggested that the onset of intense shock may trigger the brain into producing a large amount of one or more of the endorphins and that the sudden release of these natural pain killers may put the organism into a trance-like state.

Selye (1956) describes the initial reaction to impact as the 'alarm reaction': body and mind are in a state of shock; temperature and blood pressure drop; tissues swell with fluid; muscles lose their tone; thinking is unclear and ability to log information into long-term memory may be affected.

When realisation dawns that the individual is living through a disaster she/he tends to focus on her/himself. Accounts of people caught in crumpled railway carriages or collapsed buildings illustrate how they first become aware of their own condition and then gradually realise that others are involved.

Psychophysiology has several theories to offer about how people react to an unexpected event. Generally, they consist of an alarm reaction when bodily defences are mobilised, followed by a gradual return to a resting state. The problem in a disaster impact is that the unexpected event produces a situation which is not only fear invoking and exceedingly unpleasant but prolonged.

Fear

The psychological state during impact is one of very high arousal, accompanied by extreme fear, with orientation mainly towards protection of self. As the initial alarm reaction passes, the individual scans the surroundings for clues about the level of danger. This is the beginning of the inventory stage.

Fear is the dominent response when threat to survival is imminent, and the physiological concomitants of the accompanying arousal are racing heart, dry mouth, a feeling of tightness inside, and tenseness in the muscles. Such a state is costly to bodily resources. Homeostatic or self-regulating mechanisms eventually reduce these responses, but we do not necessarily stop feeling afraid. The fear can be fairly generalised for the safety of self and others and also specific about further injury or death.

Helplessness

The feeling of helplessness is also a major psychological component of the experience. We spend our lives seeking to control what happens to us and to a large extent succeeding. Caught in a disaster, we who decide when to get up, when to eat, when to work, when to play and when to sleep, now lie trapped in a collapsed building covered in rubble and debris, or caught below deck in a capsized ferry. Raphael (1986) says:

> the disaster continues, the person is inevitably confronted with his own ineffectiveness. Fear rises, as do feelings of helplessness, which may lead to further fear . . . But the helplessness predominates; and it is the quality, intensity and experience of helplessness that is a major factor in the imprinting of the impact.
>
> (Raphael, 1986: p. 59)

People often report a strong sense of abandonment which is in itself terrifying and the yearning for rescue can become desperate.

Loss

There are many kinds of loss and no one loss ever occurs in isolation. The kinds of loss experienced during the Impact and Inventory stages are many; some are transient, but many are not. The transient losses may include loss of freedom, loss of mobility, loss of the planned immediate future. What usually remains are memories of the distant past, pre-impact, and the experience of now. Recent past may be lost as consolidation of the recent memory may have been disrupted by head injury or shock. The psychology of loss and bereavement will be discussed in the final section of this chapter.

The psychology of disaster

Disaster behaviour

The variety of behaviour people caught up in disaster impacts exhibit has been well-documented. It ranges from flight and escape to protective postures such as shielding face or head, shielding others, for example, covering a child with your own body, family-oriented behaviours: searching for loved ones, affiliative behaviour: staying close to others or huddling together, and heroic behaviours of putting safety of others before safety of self.

Panic

Weisaeth (1983) defined panic as, 'disorganised behaviour marked by loss of control'. This definition covers both the frantic behaviour of trapped people, as well as uncontrolled, agitated and inappropriate flight in the face of threat.

Raphael (1986) asserts that, contrary to popular belief, panic is rare and limited to a small percentage of people and situations. Quarantelli (1954) specified some of these situations: the presence of immediate danger; when escape routes are blocked or about to become blocked (e.g., on a burning aircraft, see Chapter 11); when a person is isolated and unable to communicate with other people and does not know what to expect. These three situations, however, are not rare in disaster and emergency situations and so other factors such as personality and coping styles are also likely to be relevant.

Two points about panic are worth thought. First, not all panic behaviour is non-adaptive, as uncontrolled irrational flight may lead to escape and safety. Second, panic is nonsocial, even antisocial, as the panicking individual has no thought for the safety or needs of other people caught in the same situation.

Disaster syndrome

Tyhurst (1950) suggested that between 20% and 25% of people caught in a severe disaster may appear dazed, stunned, apathetic, and passive. They sit or stand immobile or wander aimlessly, unaware of surroundings, danger, or the presence and needs of others. Such a constellation of behaviours has been called a disaster syndrome. Usually the behaviour is transient, but it can last for several hours. The disaster syndrome then appears to be replaced by appropriate behaviour, but it may be followed by hyperactivity.

Survival behaviour

A number of psychological factors are involved in survival. An important one appears to be our attachment to other human beings. Struggling alongside and cooperating with someone else is altogether different from struggling alone. Pro-social behaviour such as helping and sharing appears to dominate and resources may be combined for the good of both so long as the survival of both remains a possibility.

People caught up in such situations often report a determination to be reunited with their loved ones and this probably contributes to the most important survival factor, the will to live.

Many people respond to a disaster impact by praying, even those who have never believed in a benign deity will beg a power outside themselves to save them. Others report bargaining with God or fate: 'Just get me out of this and I'll . . .'.

Alongside prayer is the response of hope, defined possibly in this situation as an 'active longing for rescue'. Dimsdale (1974) in a study of concentration camps concluded that, 'hope functions to control mood, by promoting the belief that what is happening cannot last'.

Psychological factors in rescue and remedy

Stress in the victims and helpers

Much of the work on stress treats the experience of stress as having a long time-span. In disaster situations the stressors are acute, both in terms of severity and time, but the response to them may have a very long time-span indeed.

Psychological research into stress has been going on for at least three decades during which a number of explanatory models have been developed. Selye (1956) saw stress as a 'nonspecific physiological response in which an individual reacted to a stressor first, with alarm and then resistance'. If the stressor continued, resistance eventually deteriorated as bodily resources were used up, and in extreme cases, collapse and death ensued. Selye believed that the stress response did not depend on the nature of the stressor and represented a universal pattern of defence reactions serving to protect an individual and preserve her/his integrity (General Adaptation Syndrome).

In contrast to Selye's response-based model of stress, stimulus-based models saw the characteristics of the stressor as all-important and used analogies with Hooke's Law of Elasticity:

> If the strain produced by a given stressor falls within the 'elastic limit' of the material, when the stressor is removed the material will return to its original position. If the elastic limit of the material is exceeded, permanent deformation results.

People have a built-in resistance to stressors, but when their elastic limit is exceeded permanent damage, physiological and psychological, may result. Measuring the load or stressor would give a measure of the stress experienced. One problem with this is that it follows that an undemanding situation cannot be stressful when often the reverse is true.

Recent theories incorporate parts of both these types of model but see as the important element the individual's transaction with her/his environment. Such theories see the individual as perceiving, reasoning, responding and monitoring the effects of responding and responding again and so on.

Two major components in any stress situation are the actual demand being placed on an individual and her/his actual capability to cope with it. Cox and McKay (1976) suggested that important components of the situation are the individual perception of the demand (perceived demand) and her/his perceived capability. Demand is usually seen as a feature of the external environment, but Cox (1978) points out that an individual's psychological and physical needs give rise to an internally generated demand as well. The individual makes a cognitive appraisal of the match between the total demand (external and internal) and her/his capability. If the perceived demand is not matched by the perceived capability, stress responses are triggered which can be physiological and behavioural and accompanied by changes in emotional experience. These responses act to try to reduce the imbalance between perceived capability and demand.

One way of helping people to cope with stressful situations is to increase their actual capability. Rescue workers, for example, are trained in different rescue procedures; firecrews train by learning fire fighting techniques in practice trials. Such training also serves to reduce the perception of demand by giving them experience of working in blazing buildings and so on.

It also alters the balance in the demand for the two types of information processing described earlier in the chapter. Much of the training of paramedics in rescue teams involves learning to follow certain guidelines automatically, so that the number of options they have to consider, and therefore the amount of the slower controlled information processing they have to do is minimised. The blazing wreckage of a motorway crash is no place to work out how to set up an IVI. The ambulance personnel must be able to do this speedily and confidently; that is what training is for. This not only helps to prevent potentially fatal errors but also reduces stress amongst the helpers.

It is fairly easy to see that once you are trained, your potential for being a bystander is considerably reduced. If you have already seen this type of emergency, you know you know what to do and how to do it, and you have accepted the responsibility for helping before. Evidence of this can be found in the media reports; notice the number of off duty policemen, firemen, nurses and doctors who are involved in emergency rescues.

An important point about response to stressful situations is that if a situation demands too much of us, and we have not realised our own limitations, we will work on without being stressed until it becomes obvious that we can no longer cope. Having collapsed, however, it becomes clear that a massive overdraft has been run up in bodily resources. Again, part of training and rescue team management has to be to prevent rescuers getting into this state. Theatre teams in hospitals must be protected by good management from this sort of situation, see Chapter 9.

Part of the psychological response to stress suggested by Cox and McKay (1976) is cognitive defence. This may take the form of denial of which there are two types. Denial of facts involves distortion of reality and this may be what is happening in the transient disaster syndrome described earlier. The other is denial of implications, ignoring the long-term negative consequences of actions or events; this may be what happens in rescue workers who work until they drop.

Victims of disaster are in highly stressful situations and, as far as the victim is concerned, the most important thing is to take action to reduce the demand as she/he perceives it. Clearly the long-term goal is to remove the actual demand by removing the victim from the disaster area but this may take time. Another action then may be to administer painkillers and/or tranquillisers to reduce both the internal demand and alter the perceived demand.

Psychological first aid

Raphael (1986) lists the components of psychological first aid appropriate in the rescue and remedy stages of disaster and emergency situations. These include:

Comforting and consoling by holding and touching can convey the emotional meaning of care more than any words. 'Being with' provides an anchor point for the victim whose world has been torn apart and points of reference destroyed.
Protecting by staying with dazed and stunned people may be sufficient to protect them from further harm.
Care of physical necessities by treating injuries and providing warmth, protection and food are interwoven with the first two.

First aid also involves goal orientation for disoriented individuals such as helping them work out what to do next, helping to search for or providing information about families, and providing emotional support if victims have to identify dead relatives or friends. Some people will express their feelings spontaneously. Raphael (1986) says this should be accepted, but always with the idea of helping the victim to reconstitute her/his defences and regain control until a more secure emotional situation is reached in which the experience can be worked through.

Re-establishing a sense of security can be started by providing some structure and timetable within the victim's disordered environment. Even within the first few hours, linking victims with other victims can permit the development of supportive groups where sharing and talking through experiences can happen and new developments can be interpreted together. (See Chapter 9 to see how this worked for survivors of the 1982/1983 IRA bombing campaign.)

Some victims may show extreme psychological reactions such as acute manic episodes or depressive withdrawal, intense anxiety or panic reactions. In the short-term, such people may be helped by tranquillising medication.

Raphael (1986) completes the list of components with a plea for 'psychological victim' identification, particularly for people showing extreme psychological reactions who may need prolonged professional help. The importance of victim identification lies in enabling the possibility of follow up and linking people with systems of support which should continue in the recovery phase.

Bystander or helper?

Amongst the untrained public, why do some people come to see and stay to help, whilst others only come to watch? The psychology of bystander intervention is a very interesting one and work on it really began in 1964 when the case of Kitty Genovese became the stimulus for research. She was stabbed to death at 03.00 hours on 18 March 1964 only a few yards from her New York apartment. What caught the headlines was that the investigators discovered that at least 38 of her neighbours had gone to their windows to see what was happening; 38 people who had done nothing. Sadly, similar instances are not uncommon these days.

What factors come into play in such situations? Latané and Darley (1969; 1970) identified the following:

> An emergency involves threat or harm and very few positive payoffs for anyone who takes even successful action.
> People have little experience of emergencies as they are rare events.
> One emergency can differ very much from another requiring very different action from a witness (viz., drowning, fire, assault).
> Emergencies are unforeseen so witnesses have to cope without forethought or planning.
> An emergency requires instant action with no time for considering alternatives and this is very stressful for a witness.
>
> (Latané and Darley 1969; 1970)

Rather than condemning bystanders for not acting, Latané and Darley (1970) considered that the bystander in an emergency situation was put in an unenviable position and that it was surprising that anyone ever intervened.

Latané and Darley (1970) developed a model of the emergency intervention process in which they suggested that when someone is confronted with an emergency there are a number of decision points which she/he must pass if she/he is going to intervene. Only one set of choices will lead to action. First, she/he must *notice* the situation, *interpret* it as an emergency, and then decide whether she/he has the *responsibility to act*. If yes, the next decision is *what to do and how to do it*. The options here are direct intervention or indirect intervention (get help). At this point, the amount of danger facing the bystander and her/his perceived capability are major determinants in deciding what to do.

The intervention process is most likely to break down in either the interpretation or assuming responsibility stages. Latané and Darley (1968) suggested that in an emergency situation bystanders may just stand and stare and do nothing, but in fact at this stage they have not decided if there is cause for concern. They called this a process of 'pluralistic ignorance'. For example, how long did it take people in Hungerford to realise what was happening? Until somebody does something, each bystander sees only apparently calm people doing nothing. The other bystanders are acting as sources of normative feedback (to act unconcerned) and informational influence (there is no emergency). As no one looks worried, it cannot be an emergency so no one assumes the responsibility to act, and no one helps.

Another important idea is 'diffusion of responsibility'. We tend to assume a responsibility to help each other and to assume that others share this responsibility. The more bystanders there are, the less is each individual's responsibility. We cannot believe, therefore, that someone has not already helped by summoning the emergency services. In addition, other people have more relevant skills: 'I cannot swim'; 'I am not a nurse'; 'I cannot stand the sight of blood'. The costs in guilt and shame of not helping are reduced by assuming that the responsibility for helping is shared by everybody else who is watching.

Social psychology experiments have shown that people are far more likely to help in an emergency situation if they know that they are the only person there who could help (Latané and Rodin, 1969). Whether they help or not is strongly influenced by whether other people appear nonchalant about the event that is taking place (Latané and Darley, 1969). Ambiguity, pluralistic ignorance, and diffusion of responsibility are important factors in making a decision to help.

Other workers have approached the issue from a different angle, suggesting that witnessing an emergency is a psychologically and physiologically arousing event. In the Arousal Cost/Reward Model, Piliavin *et al.* (1981) suggest that if helping is to occur, the bystander must interpret the arousal being experienced as caused by the victim's distress rather than by anything else. In which case, arousal can be reduced by helping.

Psychological factors in recovery

Loss and bereavement

In the inventory after impact phase and during the rescue phase, the dead are counted. No account of psychological factors in disasters can be complete without a consideration of the facing up to death and the meaning and consequences of the loss of loved ones. Many volumes exist on the subject in the psychological literature. Authors well worth reading are Bowlby (1981), Tatelbaum (1981), Kubler-Ross (1975) and Hinton (1967).

When an individual loses a loved one, it is sometimes easy to forget that she/he is experiencing not one loss but many. Loss of a husband or wife, for example, may involve not only the loss of the person you loved the most, but also your dearest friend and the loss of shared memories, opinions, attitudes and hopes. It can also mean loss of income, loss of social status, loss of friends and acquaintances to which one had access through one's partner, and loss of familiar valued activities which you always did together and loss of the planned future.

Such a loss in itself is its own disaster for the individual, and the experience of shock and disorientation, the sense of unreality and disbelief are common to the two situations.

People involved in disasters may be physically injured and have to face loss of mobility, sight, hearing, health, and independence. They may also have lost a loved one or many loved ones, friends and neighbours. All this loss may have to be faced in the absence of the people who were always there to help and support, and it may have to be faced in a new environment.

The physiological reactions which accompany the grief of loss can and often do make the individual feel ill and maybe even physically ill. These reactions together with the denial, anger, and the shame and guilt which may follow or alternate are initially outside the individual's control. In fact, ill health and the development of fatal illness is more common in bereaved people than others of the same age and sex (Parkes, 1970; Ward, 1976).

Clegg (1988) says that bereaved people perch on a strange interface between normality and psychological disorder. Previously well-balanced and resourceful people can be driven by the pain of loss and the intensity of their grief into a state of 'madness' in which they fear for their own sanity.

111

It also has to be remembered that the victim of a disaster can be found outside and far away from the primary impact area. In the case of the Piper Alpha explosion in the North Sea, those who lost their nearest and dearest were on the mainland and many miles away from the oil rig.

A real problem for such people is that in many cases they have no body to grieve over. If the last memory you have of a loved one is her/him laughing and waving, obviously in rude good health, all your expectations are that she/he continues to be. Seeing the body or the place where she/he died is an important part of coming to terms with the fact that the person has gone from you and will not return. Some of those who lost relatives and friends in *The Herald of Free Enterprise* ferry disaster or the Piper Alpha explosion had only their imagination and fantasies with which to end their loved ones' lives.

Bereavement is a process of experiences and reactions. Loss is followed by any or all of denial, anger, sorrow, guilt, shame, and the grieving process continues as old affiliations are put aside or adapted and new ones formed. Gradually the loss becomes accepted and the individual begins to assimilate the fact of it into her/his life and to adapt to it, eventually taking on new experiences and challenges as recovery progresses.

Unfortunately, these days there are considerable pressures to collapse the grieving and mourning process into the shortest possible time. The Victorians appear to have understood the value of the mourning period so much better than we do today. The pomp and ceremony associated with death, black horses and hearses, funeral processions and mourning clothes marked the social acceptability of grieving. Even elaborate monuments proclaiming the virtues and achievements of the departed provided a place where it was acceptable to weep. These days we spend 20 minutes at the crematorium, have a few days compassionate leave from work, live through an agonising fortnight or so when people put up with us talking about the departed (but are much more likely to tell us about their own losses) and within six weeks we are expected to have got over it and to get on with the business of living.

Those who were involved in a disaster and survived without losing relatives and friends may have lost their homes, livelihoods or have been injured. These are all losses and they too must grieve.

In addition, people caught in disasters, and particularly rescuers, see sights they never wished to see or want to see again. Having to cope with many dead bodies, which may be dismembered, mutilated or mashed can be a harrowing experience for the most experienced rescuer, see Chapter 3. These sights and memories also have to be grieved over and put aside and often help is needed to do this. How much worse is it for the 'lay person' who has never witnessed such scenes before? Consider, for example, the witnesses to the IRA bomb attack on the army bus in Omagh, 1988, which saw soldiers literally dismembered amongst the eight dead and many wounded.

Psychological aftercare

The process of adjustment to disaster experiences is a long one, and the need for reality testing by talking about the loss to sympathetic people is very real. Clegg (1988) argues that the helpers who work with people following a disaster need to have not only a good intellectual understanding of the process of bereavement but also an emotional understanding of it. They need to have faced the subject of their own death and to have some experience of personal bereavement. It is difficult to have any idea of the intensity of emotional pain without having experienced it for yourself. It is also difficult to understand the emotional and psychological reactions to the sight of disasters without some personal knowledge of them.

People caught up in disasters, who were initially just grateful to be alive, now have to come to terms with what they experienced and what they have lost. Relatives and friends can grow tired of hearing repeated accounts of their experiences and may prematurely tell them to stop raking it over: 'Pull yourself together', 'Be thankful you are alive', is the advice; and the cry 'But I still hurt' may fall on deaf ears.

Speaking of victims of crime, Kirsta (1988) commented:

> Certainly, in the majority of cases, the succour of partners, parents, close relatives and friends is integral in diminishing the severest symptoms of distress suffered by the victim ... However, many individuals soon find that the amount of time others are capable of giving may prove surprisingly limited.
>
> (Kirsta, 1988: p. 88)

Survivors of the Bradford fire (see Case Study on p. 161) have paid lavish tribute to the support groups which were set up which simply provided the opportunity to talk over and to talk out the disaster, initially with a trained counsellor, but also with others who had shared the same experience. Shared experiences appear to support affiliation between people. It is perhaps worth remembering that a hospital ward filled initially with disaster victims provides a unique social support group of people with a shared recent past. Disaster victims leaving the group on discharge from hospital lose that special support and new non-disaster admissions to the ward find a resistance to admission to the group (see Chapter 9).

Post traumatic stress disorder

A disaster victim may experience nightmares and major sleep disturbance. She/he may develop phobias of places or things associated with the disaster. Such difficulties have been referred to as post traumatic stress disorder. Stanley (1988) says in her report of the aftermath of the Whakatane earthquake:

> My husband's surgery began to fill up with patients experiencing a variety of symptoms related to shock and anxiety. People often complained of excessive tiredness, weight loss or 'just not feeling myself', and both adults and children had insomnia and suffered from nightmares.
>
> (Stanley, 1988: p. 14)

One of the problems of post traumatic stress disorder is that an individual may become unable to fulfil everyday roles and they may have to be taken over by other members of the family. Resumption of these roles later on may lead to further difficulties.

In psychotherapy, the term 'a safe "holding" environment' is used to describe what many victims need. 'Such an environment allows the victims to talk freely about their experiences without risk of being blamed, judged, criticised or have others impose their interpretations or definitions about what the victim experienced or what he or she needs or should do now' (Kirsta, 1988: p. 152).

Psychological support has to be aimed at encouraging this process of working through experiences by talking about them, recognising the emotions experienced, and accepting that they were experienced. This sometimes means that an individual has to recognise that she/he was afraid, felt guilty, panicked or thought only about her/himself. She/he has to come to understand that these were normal reactions, and accept the fact that she/he made them. By doing this she/he reinterprets the experiences, regaining some control over them, and assimilates them into her/his overall knowledge and understanding of life.

Conclusion

A seminar held in Bradford in 1987 concluded that whilst the impact phase of a disaster is managed quite well, technically, with few lives being lost needlessly, psychological needs during impact and post impact are neglected (Clegg, 1988).

There appear to be various levels of psychological care needed. The initial need for psychological first aid gives way to a need for help and support during the recovery period. Some people may require professional psychological help over a prolonged period. Many need initial help from a trained counsellor and the opportunity to join support groups. All will need the support of family and friend.

If adaptation to and recovery from a disaster and its consequences are to be facilitated, more attention has to be paid to people's psychological needs, and more planning for and provision of psychological aftercare must be made.

References

Arbous, A. G., and Kerrich, J. E. (1951). Accident statistics and the concept of accident proneness. *Journal of the Biometric Society*, **7**, 340–429.

Bowlby, J. (1985). *Attachment and Loss. Volume 3: Loss – Sadness and Depression*. Penguin Books, Middlesex.

Clegg, F. (1988). Disasters: Can psychologists help the survivors? *The Psychologist*, **1**(4), 134–5.

Cox, T. (1978). *Stress*. Macmillan, London.

Cox, T., and McKay, C. J. (1976). *A Psychological Model of Occupational Stress*. Paper presented to Medical Research Council Meeting: Mental Health in Industry. London.

Dimsdale, J. J. (1974). The coping behaviour of Nazi concentration camp survivors. *American Journal of Psychiatry*, **131**, 797–7.

Fraser, D. C. (1958). Recent experimental work in the study of fatigue. *Occupational Psychology*, **32**, 258–63.

Hebb, D. D. (1955). Drives and the CNS (conceptual nervous system). *Psychological Review*, **62**, 243–54.

Hinton, J. (1967). *Dying*. Penguin Books, Middlesex.

Hunt, E., and Lansman, M. (1986). Unified model of attention and problem solving. *Psychological Review*, **93**, 446–61.

Janis, I. L., and Mann, L. (1977). Emergency decision making: A theoretical analysis of responses to disaster warnings. *Journal of Human Stress*, 3, 35–45.

Kahneman, D., and Triesman, A. (1984). Changing views of attention and automaticity. In *Varieties of Attention*. R. Parasuraman and D. R. Davies (eds). Academic Press, New York.

Kay, H. (1971). Accidents: Some facts and theories. In *Psychology at Work*. P. B. Warr (ed). Penguin Books, Middlesex.

Kirsta, A. K. (1988). *Victims Surviving the Aftermath of Violent Crime*. Century Hutchinson, London.

Kliman, A. S. (1976). The corning flood project. Psychological first aid following a natural disaster. In *Emergency and Disaster management: A Mental Health Sourcebook*. H. J. Parad, H. L. P. Resnick, and L. P. Parad. Charles Press, Maryland.

Kubler-Ross, E. (1969). *On Death and Dying*. Tavistock Publications, London.

Latané, B., and Darley, J. M. (1968). Group inhibition of bystander intervention in emergencies. *Journal of Personality and Social Psychology*, 10, 215–21.

Latané, B., and Darley, J. M. (1969). Bystander apathy. *American Scientist*, 57, 224–68.

Latané, B., and Darley, J. M. (1970). *The Unresponsive Bystander: Why Doesn't He Help?* Appleton-Century-Crofts, New York.

Latané, B., and Rodin, J. (1969). A lady in distress: Inhibiting effects of friends and strangers on bystander intervention. *Journal of Experimental and Social Psychology*, 5, 189–202.

Miller, G. A., Gallanter, E., and Pribram, K. H. (1960). *Plans and the Structure of Behaviour*. Holt, Rhinehart and Winston, New York.

McDermott, W. V. (1980). Endorphins, I presume. *The Lancet*, 2, 1353.

Piliavin, J. A., Davidio, J. F., Gaetner, S. L., and Ward, R. D. (1981). *Emergency Helping*. Academic Press, New York.

Parkes, C. M. (1970). The psychosomatic effects of bereavement. In *Modern Trends in Psychosomatic Medicine*, O. W. Hill (ed). Butterworth, London.

Perry, R. W., and Greene, M. (1982). *Citizen Response to Volcanic Eruptions: The Case of Mount St Helens*. Irvington, New York.

Powell, W. J. (1954). An introduction to the natural history of disaster (unpublished). Cited in *Bushfire Disaster: An Australian Community in Crisis*. R. L. Wettenhall (ed). Angus and Robertson, Sydney.

Quarantelli, E. L. (1954). The nature and conditions of panic. *American Journal of Sociology*, 60, 267.

Raphael, B. (1986). *When Disaster Strikes: A Handbook for the Caring Professions*. Century Hutchinson, London.

Selye, H. (1956). *The Stress of Life*. McGraw-Hill, New York.

Short, P. (1979). Victims and helpers. In *Natural Hazards in Australia*, R. I. Heathcote, B. G. Tong (eds). Australian Academy of Science, Canberra.

Stanley, S. E. (1988). Living through an earthquake. *Health Visitor*, 61, 143–4.

Tatelbaum, J. (1980). *The Courage to Grieve*. Cedar Books, Heinemann, London.

Taylor, A. J. W., and Frazer, A. G. (1981). *Psychological Sequelae of Operation Overdue following the DC 10 Air Crash in Antarctica*. Victoria University of Wellington Publication, No. 27. Wellington, New Zealand.

Tyhurst, J. S. (1950). Individual reactions to community disaster: The natural history of psychiatric phenomena. *American Journal of Psychiatry*, **107**, 764–9.

Wallace, A. F. C. (1975). Human behaviour in extreme situations. In *Bushfire Disaster: An Australian Community in Crisis*, R. L. Wettenhall (ed). Angus and Robertson, Sydney.

Ward, A. W. N. (1976). Mortality of bereavement. *British Medical Journal*, **1**, 700–2.

Weisaeth, L. (1983). *The Study of a Factory Fire*. Doctoral Dissertation. University of Oslo, Norway.

8

Disaster: the media and the emergency services

It is a fact that disaster is news, and in a free society the media have a duty to report such major events. It would be an unhealthy and undemocratic society if the media did not have this freedom. However, if freedom is not to be abused, it must be accompanied by responsibility. In the case of disaster situations, it could be argued that this includes the responsibility of not hindering the rescue and relief operation, thereby jeopardising life and increasing the suffering of the survivors. It also means not exploiting the survivors for the sake of sensational news coverage when the real aim is to boost newspaper circulations or viewing figures.

At the scene of a disaster, and subsequently in hospital, the interests of the media and the emergency services are often very different. The media have a story that they must cover and relay back to their head offices for transmission or printing, while the emergency services are seeking to save life, relieve suffering and bring the situation under control. Despite these differing aims, it is possible for the two to coexist and even to do so in such a way as to be mutually beneficial.

If readers doubt the news value of disaster situations, look at the accounts given in the second part of this book of some recent disasters. A press corps of 100 is average. Television coverage will not only be from the British Broadcasting Corporation (BBC) and Independent Television News (ITN), but European and even American television crews will descend on the scene within a matter of hours.

If the Hungerford shootings are taken as an example, within 15 minutes of the story breaking, BBC West had three crews on the road from Bristol, BBC South sent a crew from Southampton, a further crew was sent from London, while yet another BBC crew was in a helicopter covering the whole area. A total of six camera crews from just one station.

Major events such as Hungerford or the Zeebrugge ferry tragedy involve seven or eight television news stations on scene. Each television crew consists of technicians, cameramen, a producer and production assistants, and a journalist to present the story to the camera, perhaps as many as eight people to a team. Fortunately radio coverage is much more limited, perhaps only one reporter with a tape recorder. In addition, there are also the representatives of the press; local, national and international. The emergency services therefore have to be able to cope with press corps of this size when drawing up plans, both in the field and at the hospital later.

Before considering how the emergency services and media may help each other to function properly, some of the difficult ethical questions concerning limits and privacy need to be considered. A good starting point is that the broadcasting companies concede that there are limits beyond which the camera and microphone should not transgress. Guidelines are laid down for crews in advance, within which they are expected to operate. However, in the real situation, it is the cameraman in the field who is the guardian of good taste. He alone is the person who can take the decision to point the camera away from some scene, or to turn it off altogether.

The importance of the cameraman's role in this respect is enhanced when the workings of an average newsroom are considered. Once a story has been received by the news desk and a decision reached that it is to be covered, a crew is dispatched immediately with the aim of getting pictures of the event as soon as possible. It is in the nature of events that the first pictures will be the most dramatic and, as television is a visual medium, pictures are of prime importance. The result is that the camera crew may arrive on scene with scant information to work on, events perhaps still in their most confused state, and often ahead of any journalist. In addition, they are very aware of the deadlines for the next news bulletin. This all conspires to put a lot of pressure and responsibility on the crew.

In theory, there is a second line of defence when it comes to good standards and taste, and that is the editing process that goes on before broadcasting. However, such is the immediacy of news coverage, there may be little or no time for careful consideration before broadcasting, leaving 'good taste' very much in the camera crew's hands.

The Hungerfood shootings give a good indication of the sort of time pressures that newsrooms work under. Geographically, the incident took place on the borders between the regions covered by BBC West (Bristol), BBC South (Southampton), and London. The story first came to the attention of the newsroom in BBC West at 14.45 hours. All three available crews were dispatched to cover the story, leaving Bristol at about 15.00 hours, heading for Princess Margaret Hospital, Swindon (61 km, 45 miles from Bristol), Hungerford and the garage near Hungerford where Michael Ryan had attempted to shoot the cashier.

The material gathered by these crews had to make the deadline of the main six o'clock news. It takes an hour to get to Swindon from Bristol, and an hour to get back with the video tape for broadcasting. The crew had to find the hospital, park their vehicles, find out what was happening and then get a story together, knowing that to make the transmission deadline the video tape had to be away from Swindon well before 17.00 hours. The reporter, Grant Mansfield, had only 20 minutes after arrival in Swindon to assess the situation and get his first piece together for the news. The other crews had to get their material together on a similar timescale. Needless to say, there was no time to go through and carefully edit the tape before transmission on the main news! Meanwhile, the BBC had to get the technology out to Swindon to do a live outside broadcast from the Princess Margaret Hospital by 18.30 hours featuring the reporter talking to camera.

Up to the early 1980s, news coverage was all on film, therefore there was time while the film was being developed, say an hour or so, to deliberate the pros and cons of what to show. The advent of video tape now means that news transmission can be instantaneous and, given the pressure of current affairs, it has to be. Newsrooms simply have not the luxury of time to consider and edit tape of a major event such as a disaster. Editing is very much in the hands of the front line cameraman.

Similarly, it is up to the journalist to exercise self-discipline and discretion in going about his/her work on scene, such as seeking interviews with survivors and relatives. Fortunately, the broadcasting media do, by and large, try to operate within responsible policy guidelines. However, when considering the press, there is evidence that this is not always the case.

Whilst the more serious newspapers do exercise restraint, it is a fact that the tabloid's pursuit of what are euphemistically called 'human interest stories', and their sensationalist style of writing, leads them into areas of reporting that cause serious problems for both emergency workers and the survivors and their families. There are allegations of reporters from such papers harrassing staff and survivors, and even of attempting to obtain information by deceit. It is a crucial aspect of hospital A&E policy that no detailed information concerning survivors should be given over the telephone (How do you know the person on the telephone is the relative that they claim to be?), while the need for correct staff identification cannot be emphasised enough. After all, what is there to stop an unscrupulous reporter 'borrowing' a white coat and getting their story by pretending to be a member of the hospital staff?

In this context, it should always be remembered that the police can remove any member of the press who, in the opinion of the emergency services, is getting in the way or being a nuisance. This is a last resort, but it is available if needed.

The majority of the press try and do their job and play by the rules. However, so fierce is the competition between the tabloids for circulation that there are very strong pressures indeed to try and get a different slant on the story behind the more factual, analytical style of the quality newspapers or broadsheets as they are sometimes known. This different slant is usually a personal one. There is greater interest therefore in producing a story structured around the experiences of individual survivors and also the emergency personnel. This in turn leads reporters from the tabloids to be more interested in personal interviews, and if access to key personnel is officially denied, this may lead to the use of other tactics to get a story.

This latter point of course applies to all the media because they have a duty to report the truth. If the authorities attempt to shut out the media completely from a disaster, then the media will understandably be very concerned and use whatever means they can to get the story. In the process, they may well infringe limits of privacy and get in the way of the emergency services. It is therefore making a rod for the emergency service's back to attempt such a news blackout. Controlled cooperation with the media will reduce the pressures to resort to more dubious and troublesome practices to obtain information, leading to less friction and generally making life easier for everybody. The circumstances must be extreme before such a blackout could be justified, and if the gravity of the situation were indeed so severe, then the media would be more likely to cooperate if an explanation was given.

The press differ from broadcasting companies in one important respect; newspapers usually have a political bias and this is generally of a right wing nature. A glance at the front page headlines any morning will show how such a political bias affects the reporting of news stories, and disasters are no exception. Large scale inner urban unrest or major industrial disputes involving large groups of pickets and demonstrators are highly political situations and a paper's reporting of the event will vary with its political persuasion. In dealing with reporters from the press, spokespersons should always bear in mind the political context that their words may be taken in and how quite innocently a controversy may be sparked off by an unguarded comment which is picked up by the 'shock horror' school of right wing journalism.

Having considered some of the ethical issues involved, some of the practical points of how the media and emergency services can help each other are discussed below.

The broadcast media are able to distribute a great deal of information to a lot of people very quickly. In the event of a major environmental incident, such as a leak of toxic gas or radioactive material, it may be necessary to evacuate a large area quickly. Broadcasting via local and national television and radio can get the message across very quickly to those people at risk.

A further vital use in this situation is to minimise panic. Nothing causes panic quicker than unsubstantiated rumour. Correct use of the media can allow the authorities to calm down a situation by reassuring the population about risks and the reasons for evacuation. Difficult ethical decisions may arise concerning how much to tell the population, as it may appear best to withhold some information for fear of actually causing panic.

Similarly, in the case of a major road traffic accident, the radio in particular may be used to warn motorists to avoid a certain area or turn off the motorway at a certain junction. This facility reduces chaos, makes access for emergency vehicles easier, and reduces the risks of secondary accidents being caused by traffic piling into the congested area at speed.

News broadcasts supplement the call-in system for bringing off duty staff into the hospital to deal with a major incident. On hearing the news most staff make their way to hospital immediately without waiting for a telephone call. Experience has shown that, so effective is this channel of communication, usually there are more staff reporting for duty than needed!

When news of an incident breaks, understandably, there are large numbers of people concerned that their relatives may be involved. The first reaction is to telephone the hospital to where the casualties are being evacuated, leading to a jammed switchboard in a matter of minutes. Press interest can have the same effect. A vital role of the broadcasting media is to publicise a casualty bureau telephone number where details of casualties and survivors may be obtained. Such a bureau is usually run by the police and, apart from informing distressed relatives whether their loved ones are indeed involved in the incident, it will take a tremendous load off the hospital switch-board.

To illustrate the scale of such an operation, the Metropolitan Police Casualty Bureau has 30 telephone lines and in the event of a disaster is manned by volunteers, mostly women police constables (WPCs). During the aftermath of the King's Cross St Pancras underground fire, it is estimated that the bureau handled calls at the rate of well over a thousand per hour. To deal with such a flood of calls, a computerised stacking system is used. Therefore, callers should not ring off as their call will be answered in its turn, however long it takes. It can be seen that early identification of the dead and survivors greatly facilitates the work of such a system.

The distribution of casualty information is greatly facilitated by the use of pre-recorded tapes. The Metropolitan Police bureau has the facility to play four one minute tapes giving casualty details, etc., to 250 incoming calls at once. However, such tapes must be regularly updated.

Telephone calls are not only made by relatives. Local newspapers and international news outlets routinely check the casualty lists to identify any people from their own town or country who may have had the misfortune to be involved. If, for example, a family from Whitehaven in Cumbria have been involved in an aeroplane crash or terrorist bombing in London, that is a news story for the evening paper and local radio station in West Cumbria.

In Third World countries where blood transfusion systems are not organised on the same sophisticated lines as in the UK for example, the media are a major source of help in appealing for blood donors in the aftermath of a disaster. In the event of a large scale incident, similar appeals may still be needed in the UK despite the National Blood Transfusion Service (NBTS). The London bombings in August 1982, for example, required the Oxford and South West Regions, and the Army, each to transfer 200 units of blood to help the London transfusion services cope with the demands made on their resources.

The media are also very helpful to the police in terms of appealing for witnesses. This is particularly true in dealing with terrorist incidents such as car bombings where details of the car used may be broadcast to try and track down its movements before the bombing. Similarly, witness appeals may prove very helpful.

A more controversial link between the media and the police concerns unbroadcast video tapes of incidents that the police may wish to examine for evidence. This has recently been the cause of much controversy with the police having to use the force of the law to make broadcasting companies hand over tapes of incidents such as riots in St Paul's, Bristol, and the murder of two off duty soldiers caught up in an IRA funeral procession. This remains an area of friction between the police and the media that as yet appears unresolved.

Given that the media have a duty to report disasters and other major incidents, the ways in which emergency services may help the media are described. Such assistance is very much in the interest of the emergency services and, provided that the media have access to information in a controlled way, there should be no reason for their intrusion into the rescue and treatment areas.

Representatives of the media have got two jobs to do; firstly, acquire information, and secondly, transmit that information in the form of news.

As has already been discussed, news crews work under very tight deadlines. They therefore need to be able to identify someone who is in charge of liaising with the media immediately they arrive on scene, otherwise they will have to start asking a wide range of people for information and, consequently, hamper rescue work and casualty treatment. This requires that, both at the scene of the disaster and also in the hospital, there must be a readily identifiable press officer to take charge of this side of the operation.

The press officer can serve another valuable function besides keeping the media from inadvertently getting in the way. In seeking interviews and photographs, news crews tend to work on the assumption that if nobody says no, then they may proceed. After all, this assumption is made by doctors and nurses in treating patients everyday in hospital and the community. If a patient does not object, they are giving consent. It is up to the emergency services and the hospital authorities to say 'no' if they feel it is against the casualties' interests to be interviewed soon after the event. This situation is best handled by one person, acting on advice from the emergency services and medical/nursing staff, liaising with the press and informing them of who they may or may not speak to. If that person is readily identifiable and seen to be in control of the situation and acting fairly and consistently, i.e., has credibility as a press officer, then the problem of interviews should be resolved amicably. If not, as has been previously mentioned, the police have the power to remove anybody getting in the way!

The press officer must be knowledgeable about the requirements of the press and have the training and experience to handle the situation. While services such as the fire brigade and the police are now very aware of the need to have full-time spokespersons to deal with the media, other areas are not so well organised. It is no use the hospital delegating a member of the management staff who just happens to be on duty to deal with the press. An integral part of a hospital plan should be a recognised hospital spokesperson who has had appropriate training for their role in liaising with the media. This is no place for amateurs.

The reader is referred to the account of the Bradford City Football Club fire, Chapter 12, for an example of how a good press officer system dealt with the media successfully, leaving emergency staff free to concentrate on the casualties. On the other hand, a major complaint of the media during the Falklands War was the lack of professional liaison with the Ministry of Defence.

It is possible that several different spokespersons may be involved in a major disaster, representing perhaps fire, police and hospital, together with other large public utilities such as British Rail, a local public transport company or a private company. It would seem sensible for the spokespersons of such organisations to meet regularly to review how they might best liaise in order to try and prevent conflicting and contradictory stories from emerging. Such meetings are already under way in London in the aftermath of the King's Cross St Pancras underground disaster.

It is also important for spokespersons to have good routine relationships with local news editors, be it either television, radio or press. Regular meetings will prove invaluable, permitting accurate coverage of day-to-day stories and, in the event of a major incident, greatly smoothing and facilitating relationships all round.

If a situation is particularly serious, consideration should be given to limiting the numbers of press allowed on scene. While there is usually a fierce element of competition in news gathering, there are also times when cooperation may take place, and this is one of them. In exceptional circumstances, media personnel may be told that perhaps only one film crew, one radio reporter, one photographer and one journalist are to be allowed on scene, as more than that would hamper rescue work or endanger life in other ways. The media personnel could then be given 10 minutes to work out a pooling system and to decide who goes, a small controlled group would then be given access. In this way a truthful account of the situation may be made accessible to the media. A 60 second piece of accurate reporting can prevent hours of rumour, speculation and damaging uncertainty taking over in both the media and the public's mind.

If access is totally barred, news crews may start to resort to other means to do their job, i.e., gather information.

Arrangements to set up a press room should be made as quickly as possible. In hospitals this is easier as there is time to plan ahead. However, for the emergency services in the field, improvisation will be required as, unfortunately, prior knowledge of where a disaster is about to strike is not usually afforded. A large room will be required, well away from the A&E unit or disaster site and principal access routes. As a large number of vehicles will inevitably accompany a 100-strong press corps, thought should be given to parking facilities. It is worth spending time thinking about media vehicle parking on the grounds of enlightened self-interest. If all the vehicles are parked well out of the way, they are not blocking access routes to either the hospital or disaster scene!

The fact that television and radio have frequent news bulletins means that they need continual updating on the situation as deadlines come and go. The press usually have one deadline only, once that has been met and their story filed the pressure is largely off the reporters, not so with the broadcasters. They need frequent press conferences and updates, hourly or at least every two hours.

From time to time the spokesperson will not know the answer to a question. It is much better for the person to be honest and say that they do not know but are doing everything possible to find out, rather than allowing speculation to take over (see p. 126). It is vital that a spokesperson should talk in plain English, avoiding the use of service jargon that will either not be understood or misinterpreted.

A readily identifiable press officer and frequent updates of news in language that can be understood, coupled with reasonable access, are therefore the fundamental requirements of news gathering. The second part of the media's job, news transmission, is more in their own hands.

Given a good mains power supply, the television companies can carry on for days from their own resources with minimal disruption. A news crew is a lightweight operation, mostly the sort of equipment that can be backpacked around, working on batteries if needed. Modern video tapes can record in poor lighting conditions, removing the need for extensive lighting set ups. A news operation should not be thought of in the same terms as a major outside broadcast such as *Match of the Day* with miles of cable, huge lorries to transport large cameras and lights, etc. A news crew's equipment is all portable and carried on the backs of two or three men.

The one vital piece of equipment that is always appreciated is a telephone, preferably a lot of them. It is well recognised that one of the major weak points in a hospital disaster response is the switchboard. Therefore, everything should be done to avoid further overloading of the hospital telephones with a large press corps. A hospital plan not only needs to consider setting up a press room, but also how the press can be given access to public telephones without jamming the hospital switchboard. Commandeering pay telephones may be one solution; hospitals do have portable plug-in telephones for use on the wards. Perhaps British Telecom could be persuaded to install, as a public service, some connection points close to the press room so that telephones may be borrowed from the wards for this purpose.

Such is the news value of disasters that they prove irresistible to politicians. The current Prime Minister, Mrs Thatcher, has had a high profile in visiting disaster victims in hospital within 24 hours of the incident. It appears, therefore, that in addition to coping with the casualties, hospitals must also be prepared to handle a prime ministerial visit, with all the disruption and security implications that go with it.

While security is obviously intense around the prime minister, the question has to be asked, amongst the chaos and confusion of a hospital coping with 200 plus casualties, how effective a security check can be done at a few hours' notice? A terrorist organisation, knowing the prime minister's predilection for turning up to visit casualty victims within hours of a disaster, and knowing the exact ward to be visited (the nominated casualty reception ward in the major disaster plan) has effectively been handed a much easier target to hit. All they need to do is create the disaster in the first place with their own bomb and, if they have concealed a second bomb in the nominated casualty receiving ward perhaps some days previously, the chances of it being located are greatly reduced amongst the chaos and the very short time period for searching, if indeed a search is carried out at all. The second bomb could then kill the terrorists' prime target, not to mention the survivors, nursing and medical staff and anybody else on the ward.

The question of prominent persons visiting survivors in hospital has to be seriously examined. I believe this is no place for politicians. If the state wishes to demonstrate its sympathy with survivors, perhaps a representative of the Royal Family is more appropriate; the visit being made at least three days later when necessary security checks have been made. The present system seems to invite an organisation such as the IRA to plant one bomb as bait to lure the main target into the trap, and to have a second bomb planted, ready and waiting, in the hospital casualty reception ward.

Conclusion

In a free society the media have a right to keep the public informed of major events, and the public want to know. That is the justification for media involvement; they have their job to do just as everybody else has theirs. Liaison between services is essential for disaster planning, and such liaison must include the media as well. If each side knows what the other is trying to do, it should be possible to avoid unnecessary friction, and facilitate the smooth operation of the rescue and treatment plan, while keeping the public fully informed of events, as is their right.

Case studies

9

Terrorism: the IRA bombing campaign in London, 1982/1983

It appears to be in the nature of terrorist activity, and in particular the Irish Republican Army (IRA), that bombings are carried out by an active service unit as part of a definite campaign. Single attacks are also possible as happened, for example, in the assassination attempt on the current Prime Minister, Mrs Thatcher, at the Grand Hotel in Brighton, 1985. When an active service unit has obtained and stored sufficient explosives and detonators, and feels secure in their undercover activity, it only remains for their superiors to give the orders, and bombings will be carried out in a sequence, presumably until all the explosives have been used or the unit apprehended by the security forces and police.

As a case study, the most recent campaign carried out by the IRA in the early 1980s, culminating in the Christmas 1983 car bomb at Harrods department store in London will be discussed. In total, there were eight incidents leading up from October 1981 to the Harrods attack. The first incident was a bomb concealed in a laundry van outside Chelsea Barracks in Knightsbridge. It was detonated by remote control as a coach full of soldiers drove past, leaving two people dead and 37 injured. This bomb showed the IRA's awareness of the effectiveness of shrapnel as an antipersonnel device, as it was deliberately packed with bolts, nails, etc., to achieve this effect.

Over the next two months attacks took place against Sir Stewart Pringle, Commandant General of the Royal Marines (a booby-trapped car bomb), a Wimpy Bar in Oxford Street (Ken Howarth, a bomb disposal expert, was killed by this device), and Debenhams in Oxford Street (successfully defused). November saw two people injured by a bomb outside Woolwich Barracks, and the home of Sir Michael Havers QC, the Attorney General, attacked, but fortunately with no casualties.

A period of inactivity followed this spate of attacks until 21 July 1982, when what had been a fine sunny morning turned into a grim and bloody day for central London as two bombs, one in Hyde Park and one in Regent's Park, killed 10 people and injured many more.

The first explosion took place at Hyde Park where a bomb containing 4.8 to 9.6 kg (10 to 20 lb) of high explosive surrounded by 12 and 15 cm (4 and 6 inch) nails was concealed in a blue Austin Morris 'P' registration car. It was detonated at 10.44 hours as a troop of Household Cavalry was parading past on ceremonial dury, passing only eight feet away. By coincidence, the sister in charge of the A&E unit at the Westminster Hospital was discussing the major disaster plan with the sister from the 14 bedded casualty receiving ward that morning, even as the bomb exploded.

Eyewitnesses spoke of a fireball as the bomb exploded, and witness accounts in the newspapers the following day described seeing blood everywhere, especially covering casualties of the explosion. This is an important consideration for emergency personnel arriving on the scene of a bombing. It will all look very dramatic with lots of blood-splattered casualties, but the people on their feet, staggering around, however bloody they may look, are not likely to have sustained life threatening injury.

Ambulances arrived on the scene within five minutes of the explosion to find two dead soldiers, four other injured soldiers, and 19 civilian casualties. The picture was further complicated by the presence of many horrendously injured horses, seven of whom were dead or had to be put down, and a further nine were in need of treatment. The lesson here is that in planning for disaster, consideration needs to be given to the fact that animals may also be casualties as well as humans.

The force behind such a relatively small car bomb may be gauged by the fact that wreckage from the car was found up to 225 metres (250 yards) away, windows were blown out over a wide area, and pieces of the car were found embedded in the walls of fourth floor offices nearby. The large amount of broken glass produced by this bomb was nothing compared to that at Harrods (see p. 137), and it is a feature of bombs detonated in urban surroundings that large quantities of window glass will shower down into the streets below. This avalanche of glass causes many serious lacerations and considerably hinders rescue attempts, hence the need for protective heavy-duty footwear even when responding to an emergency in a city street in midsummer (see p. 80 on clothing for mobile teams). Considera-tion should also be given to the tyres of emergency vehicles, as an ambulance will not be a great deal of use in evacuating casualties if its tyres are cut to ribbons.

As central London contains a high concentration of hospitals, it is relatively easy to spread the casualty load amongst them. In this case, the Westminster Hospital, St Mary's, St Stephen's and Uni-versity College Hospital (UCH) were all reported as having received casualties. The decisions about the allocation of casualties to hospit-als were made by the London Ambulance Service on site, as they did for the other bombings described in this chapter.

The receiving ward at the Westminster Hospital was able to clear its 14 beds within 15 minutes. Approximately 20 casualties were taken to the Westminster, of whom three required ITU beds, only five were admitted, and the rest sent home from A&E. The ward policy calls for all patients to have their documentation kept as up-to-date as possible to facilitate speedy transfer in the event of a major incident; 15 minutes is the target time.

As it happened, the ward received its patients after theatre, which led to relatives appearing before the patients in a state of great anxiety. Considerable support was needed for the families throughout.

The five patients had suffered flash burns to the face, serious shrapnel injuries with extensive wounds, and some limb trauma. It was noted that the soldiers did not receive any chest injuries, this being attributed to the protective effect of the ceremonial armoured breastplates they were wearing. Unfortunately, the ceremonial hel-mets worn were thought to have contributed to the severity of the head injuries suffered by two other soldiers who were in ITU.

These patients spent several weeks together on the ward and developed very close links which has led to them keeping in contact years later. Ordinary patients were readmitted to the ward the following day to start to fill up the empty beds which led to tensions and anxieties. The bomb casualties found it very difficult to accept new patients as they had yet not worked out their own feelings of the horrors they had just survived.

The staff also found this a very difficult situation as, effectively, the ward was now two wards within one. There were two different groups of patients with very different needs and all under the glare of public attention. Experience suggests that after a major incident a period of several days should be left before empty beds on a receiving ward start to take patients again.

However, on the day of the bombings, as the emergency services were coping with the congestion of central London traffic and attempting to sort out the chaos in Hyde Park, they were unaware that a second bomb had been planted under a bandstand in Regent's Park where the band of the Royal Green Jackets were due to give a lunch time concert. Some two hours after the first explosion, this second bomb was detonated, killing six soldiers instantaneously and wounding 30 others.

The mobile team from St Mary's was put on a yellow alert or stand by at 13.00 hours. St Mary's was required to supply four nurses, one from A&E, and three from theatres, one of whom was to be the theatre nursing officer who would act as team leader. The team was to be completed by a senior surgical registrar and a senior anaesthetic registrar. The red alert for full action was received at 13.10 hours and Fletcher (1986) has written of how the nursing part of the team arrived at the front door of the hospital to find an ambulance waiting, loaded up with equipment by the portering staff and ready to go. Fortunately, as the vehicle moved off, the nursing leader realised that no medical staff were present.

It is a sad reflection upon the state of planning that exists for major incidents that the next stage of the mobile team call out can only be called a shambles. According to Fletcher, the nurses in the team were panicking, they had totally forgotten the contents of the panniers that they had with them, and the nurse from A&E had no idea of the plan or disaster protocol. The first doctor to put in an appearance was a medical registrar eating a bag of fish and chips who had been pushed into the back of the ambulance by the driver on the grounds that when asked if he was a doctor he said yes. The vehicle thus sped off with a nursing team that had little idea of what they were supposed to do, and a doctor with little experience in the management of trauma who was not even supposed to be on board.

Ambulance control then decided that all casualties were to be taken to St Mary's. Unfortunately, the hospital plan envisaged casualties going to the Praed Street branch of St Mary's and UCH, so not only was the team in a state of disarray, but the casualties were being taken to the wrong hospital.

The missing medical staff arrived later in a police car, together with another mobile team from another hospital. According to

Fletcher (1986), the nursing staff on the St Mary's team spent half an hour sitting on the grass contemplating the scene before being told their services were no longer required. In this period, the medical staff were asked to certify dead bodies and, at the end of this time, were visibly shaken by the appalling mutilated state that some of the casualties were in.

When the team arrived back at the hospital, the scene was one of frantic activity in A&E as resuscitation work was in full swing on the many casualties, and the theatres were desperately getting ready for what was to be a long day and night's operating. The reader is reminded of the observation on p. 72 that the staff sent out on the mobile team should have the experience to do the job they are sent to do, but not at the expense of weakening the hospital's ability to cope with casualties in vital areas such as A&E, theatres, and intensive care.

It would be unfair to be too critical of the unfortunate team from St Mary's, as I suspect this sort of situation could happen anywhere, such is the poor state of preparation and communication difficulties that exist in the NHS. They are to be commended for publishing their account of what went wrong so that others may learn from their mishaps. Fletcher herself has pointed out the fundamental error of sending the person in charge of theatres out with the mobile team when they are most required to organise theatres so that they are ready to accept the major surgical workload that a disaster will bring.

The situation in theatres was chaotic according to Fletcher because of a nonstop barrage of telephone calls from different teams of surgeons in A&E, all understandably anxious to get their patients to theatre as soon as possible. This demonstrates the need for a single medical director coordinating activity in A&E and determining priorities of treatment for casualties. At this stage, theatres had broken down into chaos as every telephone in the area was ringing with details of different patients. Fortunately, the chairman of the division of surgery gave authority to the theatre nursing officer to only accept cases that were authorised by him, thereby establishing control over the chaos.

The decision was made to work with three theatres only, as many of the patients required more than one team of surgeons. To illustrate the sort of problems likely to be encountered in the aftermath of a bombing, the first patient in theatre required skull traction for a fractured cervical spine, while the second patient was an unidentified male, suffering severe head and facial injuries, multiple wounds elsewhere about the body, and was covered in a black, oily substance that had to be scrubbed off with a rapid hand cleanser such as Swarfega before surgery could commence. The neurosurgical team found a badly mutilated skull and brain injury, the ear, nose and throat (ENT) team had to wire his fractured jaw, an orthopaedic team was involved in treating bone and joint trauma, while the multiple wounds were all badly contaminated and included pieces of shrapnel in his chest.

Other cases required the removal of nails and debris from lower limbs and faces, while extensive wound debridement was required in three further cases. Nails were removed from up to 12 cm (4 inches) deep within the body. Many of the casualties had shattered eardrums and were suffering from deafness as a result of the explosion. Most of the immediate surgery was finished by the time the night staff arrived, but one major case continued on into the night.

The police had to set up an office in theatres as officers from the antiterrorist squad began the painstaking task of assembling forensic evidence. Every piece of material recovered from the soldiers' bodies was potential evidence and had to be carefully documented. This exercise took three weeks.

It was ironic that only minutes before the second explosion, having heard of the explosion at Hyde Park, the bandmaster had searched under the bandstand but failed to find anything. The moral is simply that if there is to be a search for bombs, it would be better if the experts carried it out.

The following day brought the death of another soldier from the Household Cavalry and the reported number of casualties still in hospital was put at 22, out of the original 51 casualties. Two days after the bombing there were still four survivors in intensive care, two at St Mary's and two at the Westminster, and also the inevitable visit from the Prime Minister to hospital wards.

Two small bombs exploding within two hours of each other in central London had caused chaos and mayhem. The IRA usually claim that their targets are of a military/security nature, and therefore legitimate. The high proportion of civilians killed and injured in these two bombings seriously questions the validity of that claim. As events at Harrods and later at Enniskillin in 1987 were to prove, it should not be assumed that because of IRA claims that their targets are only military, there will not be further bombings and massacres of civilians and military personnel alike on the streets of the UK and overseas.

After a year or so of quiet in London, the IRA next struck at Harrods on Saturday 17 December 1983. Again, they used a car bomb; a blue Austin 1300 GT, the bomb being of similar size to the two used in 1982 about 11.5 kg (about 25 lb). On this occasion a timing device was used to detonate the weapon, leaving five people dead and 91 injured. The car was parked in Hans Crescent, just outside Harrods, at about noon, probably in a space that had been reserved by parking another car in it much earlier.

At 12.40 hours the Samaritans received a telephone call from the IRA stating that there was a car bomb outside Harrods, and that there were bombs in other department stores in Oxford Street. Within four minutes the Samaritans had made a 999 emergency call to Scotland Yard with this information, and by 12.49 hours details had been given to a metropolitan police radio operator to dispatch police units to the area. This message went out within two minutes, while a few minutes later another message had gone over the telegraph system to alert local police stations.

Harrods began clearing the store at 13.00 hours and, as a full-scale police operation to evacuate the area was underway, the bomb exploded at 13.21 hours. Officers from Chelsea Police Station were caught in the full blast as they were approaching the car on foot and in a police car which was wrecked. One male and one female police officer were killed and 13 others injured, one of whom was to die on Christmas Eve with severe head injuries. All were from Chelsea Police Station.

Again, the casualties were spread out among the central London hospitals and of the 90 or so casualties, 20 were still in hospital two days later, a similar sort of proportion to the Hyde Park and Regent's Park bombings. These sort of figures indicate that for planning purposes, in a situation where there is only one local hospital receiving casualties, a minimum of 20 admissions should be expected from a major incident. The most seriously injured survivor suffered traumatic amputation of his right leg and several fingers and went into renal failure. He required extensive surgery to save his left leg and was reported as being in a critical condition a week later.

The hospitals involved received their casualties and activated their plans in the usual way, although the Westminster had a ten minute start on the official notification time as one of the hospital's senior consultants was in the vicinity and called the hospital immediately to tell them what had happened. Staff at the hospital had heard the explosion and so were not surprised at the news.

The plan for the Westminster worked well with the receiving ward being cleared very quickly. The receiving ward's first casualty was an injured police officer to hold pre-operatively while theatres were got ready. This rapid movement of patients into a holding area, which the receiving ward can be used as if it is ready quickly enough, prevents tying up cubicles in A&E and greatly eases the pressure there and on theatre.

The staff were confronted with the familiar pattern of flash burns and extensive, gaping shrapnel wounds. Seven more casualties were admitted to the ward that day, with a further patient arriving via ITU later. The pattern of flash burns and shrapnel injury was repeated in these casualties. The incidence of burns in disaster victims is such that nursing staff on the designated receiving ward must be up-to-date and familiar with the care of the burns patient.

Reference has been made in Chapter 8 to the existence of a casualty enquiry telephone number run by the police to deal with major incidents. Unfortunately, the Westminster Hospital telephone number was given out by mistake in television broadcasts which led to the hospital switchboard being jammed for much of the day. Many of these calls came from overseas. Such is the potential for confusion in disaster situations, it is worth pointing out that the story that went out on the news agency wires read, '7 to 9 killed in Harrods Bombing'. By the time this story reached India, it had become '79 killed in Harrods Bombing'. The ward staff were inundated with calls from the USA, as some very garbled accounts had appeared in American newspapers and two of the casualties were Americans.

It was reported in *The Times* on 22 December 1983 that the effects of the bombing had seriously depleted stocks of blood at the Regional Blood Transfusion Centre resulting in the fact that they had to be topped up with transfers of 200 units of blood from the Wessex and South Western regions and also the Army. It would seem a worthwhile step in planning for disaster to enquire how many units of blood and blood products could be made available in an emergency by the blood transfusion service, and whether any plans exist for transfers of extra blood from other regions or emergency donor sessions.

In Chapter 7 the psychology of disaster has been discussed. It is worth reporting that a girl who survived the Hyde Park bombing, and had been a patient on the casualty reception ward at the Westminster Hospital, came forward voluntarily after the Harrods incident and offered to talk to the survivors. The horrors of such events must be talked through by the survivors and acts of courage such as these (reliving the incident for the benefit of victims of a later disaster) are greatly to be admired. Perhaps in developing post-disaster counselling services willing volunteers who have survived should be involved, as for example in patients undergoing surgery such as a mastectomy and limb amputation, to try and help support the patient.

The three major bombings described here all took place outdoors, reducing the potential antipersonnel effects of the weapons. However, as can be seen from the section on blast injury (p. 25), the bombs produced a similar pattern to that which experience suggests is to be expected with multiple contaminated wounds, penetrating shrapnel injury, ear damage and deafness, and burns and fractures predominating amongst the casualties.

In 1982/83, many people were killed and others maimed by relatively small bombs, and the disaster plan of one major London hospital was admitted to have failed, with the effectiveness of treatment depending upon individual initiatives. There is great concern amongst security services that the IRA now has substantial amounts of modern weaponry and explosives that it did not possess in 1982 or 1983, and years later is now prepared to return to London with its bombing campaign, as the attack on Mill Hill Barracks showed. If, for example, a 13 kg (30 lb) shrapnel-packed bomb were to explode in a shopping centre one Saturday lunch time, or maybe in a packed pub at 10.00 p.m., how well would your emergency plan cope?

References

Fletcher, V. (1986). When the music stopped. *Nursing Times*, **April 30**, 30–2.

10

A study of urban mob violence: the Tottenham riots, 1985

The 1980s have been marked by a series of civil disturbances on a scale not seen in the UK for many decades. Three broad scenarios are identifiable; inner urban anti-police riots, football hooliganism, and major industrial disputes. There are many similarities in these different situations, consequently, one of the more recent events, the Tottenham Riots of October 1985, will be examined in the hope that the lessons learned from this major disturbance can be applied to any such major civil incident.

Prologue to a riot

The unpredictability of disaster has already been discussed, but it has been stressed that, where possible, contingency plans should be made if risk situations can be identified in advance. Riots tend to be spontaneous events with little forewarning, although there is often a build-up in tension which the emergency services should be sensitive to. Such a build-up only needs the right trigger and a violent riot can explode in a matter of minutes.

Such was the situation on the Broadwater Farm Estate in Tottenham, London, in the first week of October 1985. This inner urban council estate had a history of racial tension, with Asian traders being the casualties of both black and white gangs. Tension between the police and some residents on the estate had a lengthy history and all this came to a head on Saturday 5 October 1985 when Cynthia Jarrett, a black woman, collapsed and died during a police search of her home which was situated just off the estate.

It is interesting to note the views of Reiner (1985) who describes the American experience of urban riots. Reiner considers that the trigger incident does not so much cause the riot as legitimise it. In other words, the riot was ready to happen and people just need a legitimate exuse to rationalise what follows. The implication of this view is that riots are not as spontaneous as might be thought. Consequently, it should be easier for the emergency services to spot trouble coming and be on alert to deal with it accordingly if they are not able to defuse the situation, which is clearly the preferable alternative.

Reiner goes on to say that rioters are often very ordinary people, not misfits or individuals unrepresentative of the community. Social deprivation alone is considered to be a very simplistic explanation; the dynamics of a riot are far more complex than saying either rioters are just bad people or that they are simply the victims of an unjust society.

It was these ordinary people who gathered outside Tottenham Police Station at lunch time the following day to protest at Cynthia Jarrett's death. At about 12.00 noon things appeared to be under control as appeals from the dead woman's family and community leaders took the heat out of the situation. However, by 14.00 hours there was a crowd of people, variously estimated at between 100 and 500, angrily protesting against the police action. Verbal abuse was hurled at the police and there was some damage to vehicles. Traffic in Tottenham High Road was stopped and a stone shattered a window at the police station.

The afternoon slid ominously towards the evening's explosion of violence when at 15.30 hours two police officers were called to The Avenue. Their car came under missile attack; pieces of concrete shattering the windscreen inflicting serious abdominal trauma on one officer.

A meeting was called on the estate for approximately 18.00 hours. The police were not invited. However, at 18.09 hours a 999 call was received with someone complaining about a group of young blacks causing trouble on The Avenue. Cautious police investigation revealed no sign of trouble so the police withdrew.

The speed with which events can develop may be judged from the fact that within 45 minutes of the first 999 call, further emergency calls were received by the police with people complaining of groups of youths throwing stones at doors in The Avenue. Police investigating these calls were violently assaulted with a hail of missiles including bottles and fire bombs. By 19.00 hours a full-scale pitched battle was developing around The Avenue, Mount Pleasant Road and Willan Road. The Tottenham riots had begun.

The opposing sides

The ensuing night of violence and murder has been portrayed as a battle between the rioters and the police, and there is much truth in this. However, there were two other very important groups involved: the ordinary people of Broadwater Farm Estate who wanted no part of any trouble but who found themselves imprisoned in their homes, or, worse still, out on the streets as the riot erupted; and, of course, the fire and ambulance services.

It is important that the personnel involved in a riot do not assume that everybody they encounter on the street is a rioter. They could simply have been taking the dog for a walk!

The rioters at Tottenham were mostly young and of mixed ethnic origins. The weapons used varied from hand thrown missiles to clubs, knives, machetes, and even empty metal beer kegs. The most worrying development at Tottenham was the use of firearms.

The emergency services had to deal with missiles which varied from stones and lumps of concrete to bottles and petrol bombs. The destructive power of these weapons was enhanced by the fact that the area involved included high-rise developments, the balconies of which were used as launching pads for rioters to drop petrol bombs and heavy pieces of concrete on to the heads of police below. Many casualties suffered head injuries from this aerial bombardment, including rioters themselves who were caught by missiles thrown from behind their own front line falling short of their intended target. Missiles also landed beyond the police front line in amongst fire and ambulance personnel.

The rioters tended to have small groups of *agents provocateurs* attempting to lure the police into ambushes. Some members of these groups wore masks to conceal their faces. Small groups were also active behind the main mass of rioters, while those responsible for using the firearms appeared out of the front line of the rioters, fired their weapons, and retreated to the safety of the crowd. It is believed that one or more shotguns were used; a .38 revolver and a .22 weapon which had been either a handgun or a rifle. A total of eight police officers and some television camera crew required treatment for gunshot wounds, fortunately none of them were fatal.

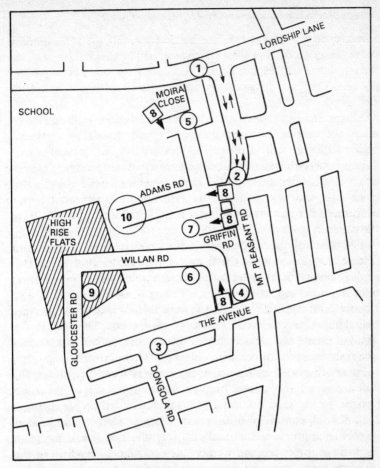

Fig. 10.1 Scene of the Tottenham riots; scale 4 cm = 250 metres.
Key: (in chronological sequence)

1 Main ambulance approach route. Casualty evacuation by same route.
2 London Ambulance forward aid post.
3 15.30; concrete lumps injure two police officers in patrol car.
4 19.00; major disturbances – missile and petrol bomb attacks on police.
5 Hour long full scale pitched battle between police and rioters.
6 Shops burnt and looted.
7 Area of shootings.
8 Coordinated large scale police counter attack pushes mob back into estate (⟵ indicates direction).
9 PC Blakelock murdered.
10 05.00; area of final resistance occupied by police.

In response to this attack, the police sealed off the area, thereby preventing rioters from spreading havoc further afield. This also had the advantage of preventing reinforcements from other areas joining the riot. Traffic exclusion zones were set up to safeguard routes for emergency vehicles.

A joint incident room directed operations thereby ensuring maximum cooperation between police, fire and ambulance services. Senior officers from all three services staffed this control. Close liaison between incident control and the hospitals receiving casualties is clearly important. On the ground, the senior fire officer acted in an independent capacity as far as fire fighting operations were concerned, but concerning security acted in the light of advice from the police.

The police were equipped with special riot clothing; an important feature of this clothing is the flame resistant material of which it is made. Senior officers are of the opinion that this saved many serious burn injuries and possibly lives amongst their personnel. The London Ambulance Service (LAS) were able to issue similar protective clothing plus helmets to some of their crews, but, due to the speed of events and the demand for casualty evacuation, many crews went into action equipped with only a protective helmet.

Police officers in riot gear look very different from the ordinary PC walking along the street. Individuals are not easy to recognise because of the essential facial protection afforded by the helmet. However, all constables display some form of identity and officers display an appropriate rank insignia. Identification should therefore be possible, providing other emergency personnel have learned the different rank insignia. Squads of riot police always have officers with them and, therefore, it should be possible for effective communication to be quickly established with the officer in charge.

On the night in question, approximately 1000 police officers were employed to contain the riot, 248 of whom reported injuries sustained during the disturbances, and approximately 25% of those who reported injuries were taken to hospital.

Baton rounds were available to the police, along with CS gas, but in the event neither were used. The effects of CS gas have been described elsewhere (see p. 41). A baton round weighs 135 g (4.75 oz) and is designed to be used at a range of greater than 25 metres, aimed below the waist. A person hit by one of the missiles would be forced to the ground with a painful blow about the same as being hit by a cricket ball bowled by a Test Match class fast bowler. However, in this case, the person would not have the benefit of pads and other protective equipment. In Northern Ireland, for example, baton rounds have been responsible for 12 deaths in 11 years. They are capable of inflicting serious injury and casualties should be treated with priority. Police are rightly reluctant to use such weapons and then, ideally, only against individuals identified as having committed or in the act of committing a serious offence.

Alongside the 1000 police officers who were attempting to contain the disturbance and restore law and order, there were also 12 fire tenders and 80 firemen, together with 15 ambulances and their crews, working to control fires and care for the casualties. Away from the riot, the North Middlesex Hospital and St Mary's Wing of the Whittington Hospital were the designated receiving hospitals.

Two hospitals were used as experience has shown it desirable to treat rioters in a separate hospital to casualties from the police and other emergency services. This principle should be adhered to, as far as possible, when the riot involves two separate groups such as football hooligans. The author remembers only too well the problems encountered at the Bristol Royal Infirmary A&E Unit when pitched battles involving Millwall and Bristol City supporters spilled over into the department.

Planning for riots should always involve the use of two A&E units, and it is clearly important that the ambulance service know which casualties are supposed to go to which hospital.

Having considered how the forces lined up on the night in question, the events of that night once a full scale riot had erupted can be discussed.

The riot

The night of 6 October has been vividly described by eye witnesses and reporters as one of confusion and unprecedented levels of large-scale violence which fully stretched the police.

Burning vehicles were a major problem for the emergency services. Thick clouds of black smoke from burning tyres obscured visibility. Petrol tanks were exploding which, apart from the hazard to those nearby, made a great deal of noise. To this must be added the shouting of the rioters, and the echo effect of this high-rise development; a combination which made verbal communication very difficult. Access to the area was also impeded by burning, wrecked vehicles.

The use of petrol bombs was a widespread feature of the rioting. A 'Molotov Cocktail', which is made by filling a pint milk bottle with petrol and stuffing a rag in the neck, is capable of covering an area of approximately eight square metres (10 square yards) with a sheet of flame on impact. Fire resistant clothing is therefore essential for any personnel deployed in riot situations; a fact that hospital planners need to consider before involving nurses and doctors in any future plans. The deployment of advanced first aid teams, consisting of police officers, in forward locations is a step under consideration by some police forces.

The rioters used any ammunition that came to hand to throw at the police and, as has been mentioned, the walkways of the high-rise flats were used to drop missiles on to the heads of the police. The effect of this is clearly shown in Table 10.1, which is an analysis of the distribution of injuries amongst police casualties. For comparison, figures are also given from other major recent riots.

Table 10.1 Percentage of total injuries for each body area sustained by police officers at recent riots (reprinted by permission of Metropolitan Police).

Area of body	Totten-ham	Brixton	Hands-worth, Birming-ham	Birming-ham v. Leeds	Luton v. Millwall	Wapping
Head/neck	24.0	13.5	23.0	25.5	37.6	22.5
Trunk/arms	38.6	43.8	33.0	18.5	21.2	28.1
Hand/wrist	7.1	8.4	18.7	0.0	9.5	9.0
Legs/feet	28.0	49.2	23.1	55.4	31.0	36.5
Other	2.3	8.6	2.2	0.6	0.7	3.9
Total	100.0	100.0	100.0	100.0	100.0	100.0

As can be seen from Table 10.1, the Tottenham riots accounted for the highest proportion of injuries to the upper part of the body. Many readers will recall watching the television with a sense of disgust as a large contingent of Millwall supporters ran riot at an FA Cup tie at Luton Town FC, ripping up the seats from around the ground as ammunition to throw at the police. Not surprisingly, this incident produced the second highest number of upper body injuries in the instances being considered here. Missile bombardment therefore accounts for a high proportion of police casualties, and other emergency personnel involved in a riot should be aware of this danger and be equipped accordingly with full protective helmets.

The Tottenham riots will, of course, always be remembered for the tragic death of PC Blakelock. There is evidence to show that groups of people are more likely to act violently than individuals (Walsh, 1985), and PC Blakelock seems to have been a victim of this aspect of human behaviour. A group of complete strangers attacked and murdered him, a large kitchen knife through the neck being responsible for his death. His death occurred as he had been working with a group of firemen: when the firemen retreated from an attacking mob, PC Blakelock was reported to have tripped and fallen, and within seconds he had been overwhelmed by a group of rioters.

The tragic case of PC Blakelock should serve as a warning to all personnel involved in riots. In the frenzy of such a situation, it is not just property that is the target of mob violence, any individual seen as a representative of the law is likely to be attacked. This raises the difficult question of how the ambulance and fire brigades maintain their neutrality, for maintain it they must. Balding (1985) described the need for neutrality by pointing out that no serious injuries had been sustained amongst fire brigade staff in Northern Ireland up to the end of 1985. However, as she points out, if police are seen riding on a fire tender, then the fire brigade will lose its neutrality, and its members will become targets for the rioters. This also applies to the ambulance service. The similarity of normal police and ambulance uniforms, especially when seen in the dark, should be noted, and steps taken to clearly identify ambulance crew as such.

The problem involved in communication at riots are clearly shown by the circumstances surrounding PC Blakelock's death. The LAS had established a forward position at the junction of Mount Pleasant Road and Adams Road. Ambulances were collecting casualties there and evacuating them by the only passable route, which was also the incoming route, from the Lordship Lane end of Mount Pleasant Road. The chaos caused by the missile debris and burning vehicles meant that ambulance crew were evacuating casualties on foot to their forward position, as vehicles could proceed no further.

At 22.17 hours the Divisional Ambulance Officer at Incident Control, working alongside the police and fire services, requested the urgent dispatch of an ambulance to the junction of The Avenue and Gloucester Road where a police constable was reported to be seriously injured. As a vehicle was dispatched, two ambulance men set off on foot to the location requested. As they and the ambulance arrived at the scene, they found that a private ambulance that had earlier been requested to leave the area had picked up PC Blakelock and left for the hospital. Subsequent newspaper reports talked of PC Blakelock going to hospital on a fire tender. The problem of private ambulances becoming involved in incidents which are under the control of the public services is clearly an area of concern and planners must take this into consideration in their future deliberations.

The ambulance service had evacuated 62 casualties to hospital by 23.00 hours, though by this time the pace was slackening allowing a reduction in the number of vehicles involved. When the final tally was made, the ambulance service had evacuated 70 casualties; 58 to St Mary's Wing, Whittington Hospital, and 12 to the North Middlesex Hospital. The incident was finally declared closed by the ambulance service at 05.53.

During the night there had been many cases of robbery and looting. Persons had used the cover of the riot for a wide range of illegal activities, while the burnt out remains of approximately 50 cars spoke for the intensity of the rioting that had taken place. In the aftermath, the police were left with the job of trying to find those responsible for the criminal activity of the night, which required detailed inquiry and evidence collection. Many of those involved suffered major stress during the night, the effects of which would only become apparent in subsequent days and weeks. Follow-up of emergency personnel and the casualties of such riots is therefore essential.

Conclusion

The Tottenham riots indicate that members of the emergency services may be murdered in riots and the use of firearms is now probable. The advance planning and joint incident control exercised by the three front line services was of great value, as was the step of splitting casualties between different receiving hospitals. Riots are no place for hospital staff, and if the deployment of hospital staff is ever considered, full protective clothing must be issued. Meanwhile, the independence and neutrality of the fire and ambulance services must be maintained in the field, as it offers their staff their best security. The efforts of all the services in Tottenham are worthy of the highest praise, as staff undoubtedly risked their lives many times to simply carry out their duty.

References

Balding, S. (1985). Fire brigades fear loss of neutrality. *New Statesman*.
Reiner, R. (1985). Harrassment of Asian traders. *New Society*, 148–50.
Walsh, M. (1985). *A&E Nursing: A New Approach*, Heinemann, London.

11

When an aeroplane catches fire: the Manchester International Airport disaster, 1985

Ian Lee

Introduction

Early in the morning of 22 August 1985, a Boeing 737 stood on the runway at Manchester International Airport, ready for takeoff. The aeroplane never left the ground as a blazing engine led to tragedy, leaving 54 people dead and requiring the evacuation of 80 more to nearby hospitals; 77 of them to Wythenshawe Hospital. In the end, however, only one of the evacuated casualties died.

This chapter deals with the major disaster plan at Wythenshawe Hospital, a plan which proved to work well, though many lessons were learned. Most of the patients the hospital had to cope with were suffering from the effects of severe smoke inhalation and related respiratory problems. Others had serious burns and trauma. How the hospital was related to the airport, the disaster plan, and a description of the hospital response to the actual disaster is discussed in general terms, and the chapter concludes with the lessons that can be learned from such a tragedy.

Setting the scene: Wythenshawe Hospital and the airport

Wythenshawe is a large suburban area some 16 km (10 miles) south of Manchester city centre, sprawling out into the Cheshire country-side. The A&E department at Wythenshawe Hospital was opened in 1973 when the new district general hospital was built. The hospital is a designated major accident hospital covering south Manchester, Manchester International Airport, a busy motorway and commuter rail network, a large oil refinery, and a substantial industrial area.

Patients are often landed at the airport from abroad and brought to A&E at Wythenshawe prior to admission or transfer home. This provides a variety of problems in the A&E department. It is also recognised that due to the international nature of the airport, language difficulties may arise in treating casualties.

The facilities of the department include a suture room, washout room, triage room, theatre, six observation beds, and examination and treatment areas appropriate to the severity of the injury, with a large resuscitation room situated near to the ambulance entrance. As part of the disaster plan, access is also available to a 12 bed '5 day ward' used for investigation and routine surgery.

The A&E department can call upon all specialities at Wythenshawe Hospital except plastic surgery, burns and ophthalmics. These problems are referred to the appropriate centres at Withington Hospital (8 km; 5 miles away) and the Royal Eye Hospital in central Manchester.

By virtue of the modern A&E facilities at Wythenshawe Hospital, a major accident plan was devised which aimed at taking the first 50 casualties from an accident, the next 50 to be taken to Withington Hospital. Withington is responsible for sending a mobile medical/nursing team to the site of the accident, while Manchester Royal Infirmary and Stockport Infirmary act as backup hospitals. Such integrated planning is essential in a large urban conurbation such as Manchester where several different health authorities are in close proximity. Regular practice is a feature of the Wythenshawe Hospital plan.

Manchester International Airport and major accident plans

Air Traffic Control (ATC) may initiate three types of messages for airport and aircraft accidents.

Aircraft accident This indicates that a crash has occurred or seems inevitable. The call would be activated by ATC and/or the aircraft captain if able. ATC would call the airport fire service using a 'crash line' and the airport telephonist using an emergency line. The airport telephonist should alert the police and the ambulance service via two private ex-directory lines, the airport duty officer and Withington Hospital. All services are then expected to activate their own plans.

151

Full emergency This indicates that an aircraft is in danger of being involved in an accident. The action should be the same as for an 'aircraft accident' state, except the message would be 'full emergency'. At this stage the ambulance service would be required to deploy six vehicles to the airport following their major accident plan, and all the emergency services would officially be at a 'stand-by' state of readiness, including the A&E department.

Local stand-by This applies only to the airport personnel as it is envisaged to cover a minor situation on site. The ambulance service and hospitals should not be informed of this state.

Wythenshawe Hospital's response to a major accident

The procedure envisages a call being received from ambulance control by the Wythenshawe Hospital switchboard operator whose role it is to inform the A&E department and senior nurse on duty.

When the hospital is put on stand-by no direct action is needed but assessment and monitoring of the situation is required, together with continual review of staffing levels and patient numbers in A&E.

When the major accident activate state is declared the hospital major accident plan should immediately be put into effect. Action cards are kept for key personnel, and on receipt of the activate instruction they take effect. For example, the sister in charge of A&E is required to:

transfer patients immediately from the resuscitation area, the six bedded observation unit, and the 12 bed '5 day ward' to the rest of the hospital;
prepare the resuscitation area for casualty reception;
inform the senior nurse for the hospital when the department and the 18 bed area is ready and proceed to the ambulance entrance ready to participate in casualty triage.

Staff call in for A&E is undertaken by one nurse using a direct line from the nursing office. To facilitate this call in, an A&E nurse register is updated at three monthly intervals and kept in the major accident manual.

While the plan involves many aspects of the hospital, it might be helpful to consider briefly the response required in the A&E unit.

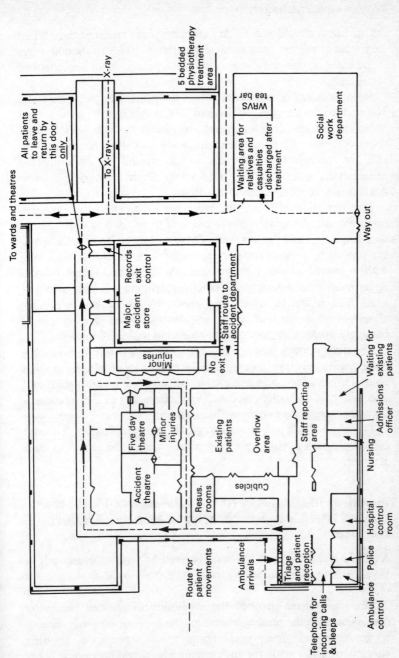

Fig. 11.1 Major accident procedure; room allocation and patient flow routes.

One nurse should assist sister with the preparation of the 18 bed area which will be used as a resuscitation bay. Intubation trays sufficient for this area are ready, pre-packed and are checked regularly.

Major accident admission packs are distributed to reception staff, 100 such packs are kept, all marked 'Major Accident'.

Major accident dressing boxes are placed in each four bedded room. These boxes have burns dressings as well as bandages, etc. IVI sets and stands are also distributed around the unit. Further preparations include making the fracture department (next door to A&E) ready to receive minor casualties.

The portering staff should erect pre-prepared major accident notices which designate areas of the unit to be used in emergencies and direct staff and patient flow. These notices are to be attached to surfaces such as walls. The portering staff are also responsible, along with a trained nurse, for obtaining IV fluids and drugs for the department from a designated major accident store in pharmacy.

As staff report to A&E, they report to the nursing office for allocation of duties and collect an identity badge. The aim is to complete preparation for casualty reception within 12 minutes.

The duty nursing officer for the hospital will also have been very busy during this time clearing the 16 bed accident admission ward ready for casualties, allocating staff, liaising with medical staff, and checking that specialist units such as theatres and ITU are proceeding with their plans to cope with casualties.

Throughout this preparatory stage, the plan emphasises that good communication is vital, and even more so once the casualties start arriving.

Nursing management on 22 August 1985: the day of the Manchester International Airport disaster

At 07.22 hours the first call was received by night nursing staff at Wythenshawe Hospital telling them to be stand-by as an aircraft was on fire.

The night sister checked the credibility of the call and, after discussion with the nursing officer in charge of the hospital, decided to do some preliminary preparations which consisted of ensuring resuscitation was ready for any patients who would necessitate being

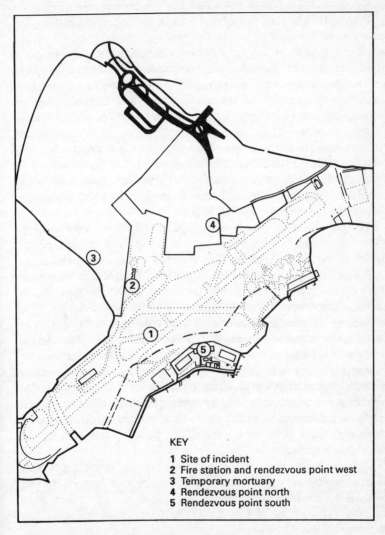

KEY

1 Site of incident
2 Fire station and rendezvous point west
3 Temporary mortuary
4 Rendezvous point north
5 Rendezvous point south

Fig. 11.2 Site of Manchester International Airport disaster.

in this area, and to prepare fluids for immediate IV therapy. Extra oxygen equipment and ventilators were available.

The day nursing staff reported on duty at 07.30 hours and were briefed accordingly. At this time, though night sister had begun preparation, the actual 'activate call' had not been received!

Day and night staff remained on duty and were waiting for the activate call when an airport bus arrived with 36 patients. The duty nursing officer then decided to activate the Major Accident Plan – though the agreed channel of communication still had not been used!

The 36 patients were quickly triaged by the associate specialist and a senior member of the nursing staff and then directed to appropriate areas for treatment. The injuries were mainly the effects of smoke inhalation, and burns and fractures caused by vacating the aircraft. Within five minutes of the arrival of the airport bus, the Major Accident Plan activated by the duty nursing officer started to show results. Doctors and nurses reported to the agreed A&E point for duty. They were allocated areas to work in by a nursing officer who acted for the A&E nursing officer.

The patients were seen, assessed again, and treated very quickly. The majority had their injuries seen to in the fracture department, which in the Major Accident Plan becomes a minor treatment area.

Pre-printed lists stating where all staff had been sent to work were kept by the acting senior nurse. On the arrival of the A&E senior nurse, duties were then relinquished by the person acting. The consultant in charge then arrived and organised treatment. The A&E senior nurse organised all staff and nursing care. The clerical and portering staff carried out their appropriate roles superbly.

Patients who had been severely burned and had acute respiratory problems were starting to arrive by ambulance – several needed resuscitation. Many were seen by other specialists (chest physicians and plastic surgeons) who had arrived in the department. At an early time after their initial treatment all the patients were seen by the appropriate specialist.

The pharmacy major accident arrangement for providing further drugs worked very well as extensive amounts of hydrocortisone, pethidine, morphine, flamazine and IV fluids were used very quickly! The stocks of nebulizers and burns dressings were sufficient.

Physiotherapists and support services were invaluable. Once many patients had been treated for their respiratory distress and oedema they were moved from the adapted 18-bed resuscitation area to the major accident admitting ward and ICU.

As deemed necessary, regular assessments of the situation were made by the A&E senior nurse and the consultant in charge. These assessments took into account patient needs, equipment, transfers and staffing levels. It proved to be a necessity to allocate nurses one patient each, with a team leader (RGN) over each group of four patients. All patients that were conscious demonstrated acute stress and emotional problems, and all in very different ways. Extensive and continuous one-to-one nursing support was necessary, apart from actual nursing.

The seventh and last ambulance arrived at 08.45 hours bringing the final patients from the scene. All these patients were assessed and treated, as previous patients had been, and nursed in the appropriate area.

A 09.00 hours the formal hospital documentation was completed. The final 'stand down' was received from ambulance control at 09.56 hours.

The patients who remained in the resuscitation area (the area designated for major accident purposes) totalled 13, all were being carefully monitored, nebulised and ventilated where necessary. It was observed very clearly that the patients who were treated with hydrocortisone for their signs of bronchial oedema improved initially, then had acute respiratory distress. Six needed to be ventilated for 48 hours, they were transferred from A&E resuscitation area to ICU.

During the time the plan was activated, the A&E senior nurse appraised the situation and reduced the staff as soon as individualised patient care permitted.

The A&E department and adapted resuscitation area was cleared, cleaned, and restocked ready for reuse, as was the major accident stock room. At 11.10 hours the department was on stand-by again for a motorway pile-up!

Other patients were treated in the department during the aircraft situation (minor injuries).

Nurses and doctors were all very much concerned and affected by the emotions of the aircraft patients and their relatives. Though every attempt was made by hospital management to control the 100 newspapermen who were around, they did become a problem at times.

Staff who had treated and cared for patients in the department so comprehensively, followed the patients' progress on the wards, and through visits, etc., after the patients' discharge. This was a very valuable exercise for the staff and certainly for the patients.

The timetable of events may be summarised as follows:

22 August 1985

Time	Event
07.13	Boeing 737 engine explodes on take off
07.22	A&E staff receive a call putting them on standy-by as an aircraft is on fire
07.23	First ambulance arrives at scene of accident
07.26	Ambulance Incident Officer arrives on site. First patients (36 in number) arrive at Wythenshawe A&E by airport bus
07.50	First press enquiry received
08.06	First ambulance arrives at A&E
08.36	Mobile medical team arrives at scene (from Withington Hospital)
08.48	Seventh and final ambulance arrives at Wythenshawe A&E
09.00	Patient documentation completed in A&E
09.56	Ambulance control declares incident stand down
11.00	Press enquiry point established
18.15	Prime Minister and VIPs arrive to visit survivors

The final casualty figures revealed that there had been 137 people on board; 54 died immediately, and one died six days later in Withington Hospital. Treatment was required by 79 passengers and one fireman. Of these 80 persons, 77 were treated at Wythenshawe; 15 of whom were admitted to ITU, with eight requiring treatment. Two patients were later transferred to the Withington Burns Unit.

Appraisal of the Major Accident Plan and its effectiveness when put into action

1 In all evaluations of major accident activate situations, the initial problems of inadequate communications seem to be present. This was the same for the Manchester aircraft disaster; the stand-by call was not upgraded to activate at the correct time. This was due to different terminology used at the airport.

2 An enquiry point for relatives, which was available proved to be inadequate – this needed more telephone lines and personnel to staff it.

3 The press were a problem for hospital management to control. (Press were not mentioned previously as the nursing response to

a major accident such as the Manchester aircraft disaster was being discussed in particular.) However, over 100 reporters proved to be a headache to senior management! There were agreed regular updates to the press jointly, and in a room away from A&E. But the press did manage to infiltrate into patient areas on two occasions and cause some upset. In future, they will be accommodated in a large committee room well away from clinical areas!

4 Signposting erected for major accident purposes in the clinical areas proved to be inadequate. This has been rectified with clear instructions on the back of each sign indicating where signs should be placed.

5 Staff identification name tags were not suitable and these have been improved. This is very important as so many extra staff of all grades and disciplines are in the clinical area and they need to be controlled and identified.

6 As envisaged, far more staff arrived in the A&E department than were necessary. The senior nurse who controls this must constantly assess the staff resources and needs, and many staff were sent from A&E to duties in their own areas.

7 There proved to be a great need for counselling and support in the case of relatives travelling together, especially where one partner was missing and the spouse did not need to be admitted. The need for close family care was paramount. Many people who had lost loved ones needed a lot of support and, in the case where hospital admission was not necessary, this could be done in someone's home until relatives had been traced. The Hospital League of Friends responded admirably to this and have set up a service for such relatives. In an aircraft disaster, passengers could be from anywhere in the world!

8 Equipment kept in a major accident store room was adequate and topping up arrangements worked well.

Conclusion

There is no doubt that, apart from the lesssons that have been learned as listed, a major accident of such proportions does test any plan. At Manchester, it worked very well. Patients were quickly documented, triaged and treatment commenced. The areas that proved to be weak in the plan have been altered.

The carers also need support after such an incident. Discussions/ support groups were set up for this purpose and were most effective. It is hoped that this chapter outlining a hospital's Major Accident Plan and its nursing response will not only have been valuable reading, but very beneficial to all who read the book.

12

A day at the football match: the Bradford City Football Club fire, 1985

Brenda Verity

Setting the scene

It was Saturday 11 May 1985 at Bradford City Football Ground. The football ground, situated on the outskirts of the city centre, dates back to the turn of the century and at the time of the fire the stands were made of timber with big spaces underneath, which over the years had become littered with rubbish.

It was a fine spring day and there was a capacity crowd in attendance as Bradford City Football Club was celebrating promotion to the Second Division in the football league and the match was to be preceeded by the presentation of the Third Division Championship Trophy. The ground itself held approximately 13 000 people, 4000 of whom were in the stand that burnt down. A high percentage of these were either very young or very old.

Bradford Accident and Emergency Unit

The A&E unit for Bradford and surrounding districts is at Bradford Royal Infirmary which is designated as the listed hospital for the Bradford district in the event of a major accident. It was built 50 years ago and no special provision was included in its design to cater for a major accident.

The A&E unit has of course been upgraded since it was built, but it is still less than adequate to deal with its normal flow of patients, and is totally inadequate to deal with an incident of this proportion. The annual casualty flow is approximately 90 000 patients. The unit at the moment consists of:

A resuscitation room which is only big enough to accommodate one patient at a time;

A room which is called the stretcher room with five trolleys separated by curtains, therefore offering very little privacy. There are no proper facilities for seeing walking wounded and they are, more often than not, also seen in this room;

There is one 'clean' theatre, one 'dirty' theatre and one recovery area. There is a 'clean' treatment room with four cubicles separated by partitions only, and a 'dirty' treatment room with two cubicles, again separated by partitions only, therefore also offering no privacy. There is a room for gastric lavage and a room which is used by the consultant and other visiting specialists for various clinics. When not in use by these doctors it is the only room available to see 'walking wounded' and is also only big enough for one patient at a time.

We aim at a minimum of eight nurses on duty between the hours of 07.45 and 21.15, of which three or four will ideally be Registered General Nurses or State Enrolled Nurses, the remaining being Students who are allocated to us for one month only. The hours between 21.15 and 07.45 are staffed by three nurses, one Registered General Nurse, one State Enrolled Nurse and one Auxilliary Nurse.

The medical cover at the time of the fire was two doctors between the hours of 09.00 and 16.00, one doctor from 16.00 to 17.00, two doctors from 17.00 to 20.30, then again only one doctor until 09.00 the following morning.

On the day of the disaster the department was unusually quiet for a Saturday afternoon, we didn't even have our usual amateur footballers in that day, it was uncanny – in fact someone remarked that this must be the lull before the storm.

The incident

The incident occurred at 15.40 hours. In the first half of the match a small fire was noticed in one of the stands, but within four to five minutes the whole stand which was packed with spectators was engulfed in flames. As a result 53 people died and 280 needed hospital treatment.

The alarm

The A&E unit first heard of the incident at 15.50 hours when we were told by ambulance control that they were bringing in a patient thought to be dead. Our policy at that time was for a doctor, accompanied by a senior nurse, to go out to the ambulance to confirm death. While we were in the ambulance doing this, the controller was saying that they had been informed of a fire at Bradford City Football Ground, a further message received from West Yorkshire Police suggested that there were approximately 30 minor casualties.

At 15.53 hours we were officially alerted by the ambulance controller that a fire had occurred, but a Major Accident was not called at that time as the number of casualties had not yet been fully ascertained. When patients started arriving minutes later, it was obvious to myself and my staff that an incident of major proportion had occurred and I rang the duty nursing officer and switchboard advising them of this. A major incident was then declared, and the Major Accident Procedure initiated.

On scene

The first notification of the incident was received from West Yorkshire Fire Control at 15.49 hours by the Ambulance Central Control. A further message was received at 15.51 hours from the West Yorkshire Police suggesting that there were some casualties. The West Yorkshire Ambulance Service's response was immediate, and the first vehicle was at the ground within minutes. By 16.01 hours Central Control had been advised by a vehicle on scene that there were approximately 25 people believed to be dead. A number of fire engines were already in attendance.

The hospital mobile team was on its way within minutes of a Major Accident being declared, but because of the close proximity of the football ground to the hospital many of the people with minor injuries that would have been treated at the scene were already making their own way to us. The more seriously injured people were already being treated and transported by ambulance crews so there was virtually nothing for the mobile team to do. The SMO and chief nurse therefore decided to return to the hospital.

The Accident and Emergency Unit

If you can picture a large department store on the first day of the sales when the doors open, that is how our entrance looked when the first group of casualties arrived, except that these were very sad and shocked people! More than 250 casualties arrived in the A&E department within one hour. They came by any means that they could; ambulance, police cars and vans, private transport, public transport and even some on foot. They were male and female, elderly and young, and had a wide range of burns. The people with superficial burns, of which there were many, had burns which seemed to be confined to the tops of their heads and their hands. This seemed peculiar to us, but we later realized that the stand had an asphalt top which was melting in the heat, and to try to stop their heads being burned people were automatically putting their hands on their heads for protection. The most serious burns were in excess of 60% of the body surface.

The sheer numbers swamped the department and overflowed into adjacent areas such as Orthopaedic, Outpatients, Physiotherapy and corridors. Our first reaction was obvious, 'how on earth are we going to cope with all these people', but once the initial flash of panic had passed and professionalism took over, we put our Major Accident Procedure into operation and everything went relatively smoothly. Expert sorting of patients must have absolute priority. We were extremely fortunate in having a team of plastic surgeons in the hospital very quickly who set the ground rules for treatments. Consultant anaesthetists were luckily having a meeting at the hospital so we had anaesthetists present equally as fast.

The Regional Burns Unit at Wakefield was alerted and the number of places they had vacant was ascertained.

The most seriously burnt patients arrived together. There were five in all who needed resuscitation and within 30 minutes they had all been intubated, catheterised and intravenous infusions commenced. Once they were stabilised they were transferred to the Regional Burns Unit. Despite being pushed to the limit, the ambulance service made vehicles available for this.

General public and off duty staff awareness was almost immediate, due to the fact that the match was being televised live. Medical and nursing staff were arriving at the hospital without being called.

On his arrival, the Director of Nursing Services (DNS) confirmed any arrangements already made by the duty senior nurse and with the information available assessed whether more nurses were required. Information regarding the function of each work area had been preprinted and the nurses were allocated to different areas. The

DNS circulated through the different areas assessing the need for extra support in manpower and equipment, and liaising with other departments, e.g., pharmacy, Central Sterile Supply Department (CSSD) and X-ray.

The ambulance liaison officer was out shopping at the time of the incident and on being called, went direct to Bradford Royal Infirmary. On arrival, she observed ambulances outside the casualty entrance and a considerable number of police and civilian cars in the same vicinity. She had difficulty forcing her way through the corridors because of the sheer volume of people. Having ascertained that the casualty radio was operational, she obtained the services of an ambulance driver to man the radio so that constant communication could be made between casualty and radio control. Excellent communications were available between casualty, the liaison officer and central control.

A 29 bedded Nightingale ward was cleared and made available so that all the patients could be admitted to one ward.

Typed instructions were issued to all medical and nursing staff, some of whom had not dealt with burn injuries for years, on how to treat the casualties and distributed to all treatment areas. 'Walking wounded' were seen and treated in the waiting areas, plaster room, physiotherapy gym or wherever available. The patients with superficial burns were treated with Terra Cortril Spray or Bactigras dressings and given outpatient appointments to return after two days, many in fact returned the next day.

Patients with burns between 5% and 10% were given analgesia and admitted to the ward for dressings. Patients with more than 10% burns were given analgesia transfused with Haemaccell and admitted to the ward for dressings.

Gradually all the casualties were dealt with and the department was cleared by about 19.30 hours. At that point we had the opportunity to take stock of the problem. We had a ward full of burned people, with some overflow on to other wards, and some of the people we had sent home would need to be treated as inpatients at a later date. It was during this discussion that the idea of early surgical intervention was developed as the option of choice.

The acute services in Bradford are on two sites – plastic surgery services are at St Luke's Hospital on the other side of the city. It was decided to empty two medical wards at St Luke's and transfer the existing inpatients from Bradford Royal Infirmary and admit patients to St Luke's direct from outpatients on their first visit. Patients who would remain as outpatients would continue to be treated at Bradford Royal Infirmary and it was decided to close the normal activities in the day ward and open a casualty burns dressing station there. Fortunately, the incident was unique, in that all the injuries were burns, with the exception of a dislocated elbow, a fractured ankle and a fractured wrist, none of which required immediate surgical intervention.

Problems at the scene

Problems occurred from the outset of the disaster. A major problem at the scene in the initial stage of the incident was the sheer volume of people funnelled into the narrow side streets in the vicinity of the football ground. Panic-stricken people were trying to vacate the ground by whatever means possible making access to the ground virtually impossible. It prevented ambulances from turning round rapidly at the incident and tended to swamp each crew with casualties upon arrival at the scene. Also, because of the volume of patients, it had not been possible to set up either ambulance control points or areas which might subsequently have been used as triage points, nor was it possible to feed in vehicles from an ambulance holding point. Staff were prevented from carrying out an appreciation of the situation and a professional assessment of the casualties. There was complete and utter confusion and chaos at the scene – crews were inundated with patients whom they were trying to load, and then they had to break off and issue dressings for immediate first aid purposes to the many dozens of casualties with whom they were confronted.

One ambulance carrying ten burned policemen was flagged down by an extremely distressed motorist who handed a child suffering from burns out of the car window into the ambulance. This child was conveyed to hospital with the policemen.

The other major problem experienced by the ambulance staff was their inability to identify a police command post or indeed their own senior officers who, at that time, were in civilian clothing.

As the ground emptied, it was soon obvious that there were a number of fatalities, burned beyond recognition, and many fused together. The bodies could not be left on an open football pitch and the city mortuary could not take them all, so there was the problem of what to do with them. Because of its close proximity to the incident, it was decided that the ambulance station would be used to provide temporary mortuary facilities. The ambulance service were then faced with the additional problem of conveying all these bodies from the ground to the depot.

At Bradford Royal Infirmary

The first major problem that we encountered was the documentation of such large numbers of patients arriving together. As it was Saturday afternoon, the clerical staff in registration were at a minimum, but having said that, had there been 5C clerks they would have been pushed to cope. Both the medical and nursing staff had to arm themselves with casualty cards and take details as they went along – so, in effect, patients were registered, seen by a doctor and, if possible, treated on the spot.

Another major problem that was soon obvious was that because patients were arriving *en masse* by whatever means available, nobody had any awareness or control over the number of patients arriving at the hospital, so the ambulance service were still bringing patients in when, had they been in full control of the situation, they would have started taking patients to back up hospitals long before they did. I in fact had to request that no more patients were brought to us.

Provision of supplies and equipment

Due to the nature and similarity of the injuries, existing stocks of Haemaccell, Omnopon, Bactigras, Terra Cortil Spray and gauze dressings within the A&E department were exhausted within a very short space of time. Initial action to restock from supplies held within the hospital was channelled through the DNS, but, as the emergency progressed, stocks had to be obtained from adjacent districts and local suppliers. The reaction to requests from the hospital was immediate and in certain instances offers of assistance were made without requests from the hospital. So it must be said that there were no major crises in obtaining supplies of any commodity, large or small, on demand.

What was a problem, initially, was keeping record of the controlled drugs used. It was decided that any patient needing analgesia, which was most of them, would have IM Omnopon. A central area

167

with two nurses doing nothing other than drawing up injections varying in doses from 5 mg to 20 mg was therefore set up. Any nurse needing analgesics for a patient went to this central area and took a syringe with the dose required. The nurses in charge of this area were responsible for balancing the amounts given and left. It was impossible to record individual names, so at the end of the day 'Fire Victims' was entered into the register and the amounts supplied, used and left were recorded. Fortunately, even after the confusion the disaster had caused, the amounts balanced.

A separate area was set up for IVIs and, again, two nurses did nothing other than run drips through, so that anyone wanting an IVI just went and got one. This was extremely useful and timesaving.

A further problem which we very soon encountered was keeping patients and their property together. All items removed were, as is standard procedure, placed in a bag and given to the patient, but I suppose due to the shocked state that the patients were in, the last thing on their minds was a bag with items of their clothing in it. They therefore became separated and, under the circumstances, it was impossible to pair them up again, so we were left with a large number of plastic bags of clothes and no owners that must have been a marathon task for someone to sort out afterwards.

Because the match was being broadcast live, the people of Bradford were immediately aware of the incident and within minutes the hospital switchboard was jammed by incoming calls. This created a very serious problem as it was virtually impossible to make any calls out thus greatly hampering the calling in of key staff and extra staff to deal with the incident. Once again, because it was a Saturday afternoon there were minimum staff manning telephones. A further two telephonists who, fortuitously, live in Bradford saw what happened and brought themselves into the hospital. Fortunately, the district ambulance liaison officer happened to be in attendance at the hospital almost from the onset. It was possible to establish radio contact between control and casualty with back up facilities between the hospitals, the central control and by the provision of the ex-directory line, all of which enabled rapid communication to be available by bypassing the main hospital switchboard which was seriously overloaded. Almost 400 telephone enquiries were dealt with during the immediate period of the emergency.

Apart from the vast number of patients, one of my biggest

problems was relatives. This was due to the fact that because the disaster received dramatic live coverage, literally as it happened, it was immediately public knowledge. I think everyone in Bradford knew somebody at that match and was obviously anxious for them and quite naturally made their way to the hospital. As we all know, everybody recognises 'Sister' and I was bombarded by all these people looking for their relatives and friends and, as news broke that there were fatalities, people were becoming hysterical or abusive as they searched for their loved ones. There was a further complicating factor in that four separate hospitals actually received casualties on the night, with two others on stand-by making it extremely difficult to draw together exactly who had been treated where.

Lessons learned

The most important lesson to be learned from this particular disaster is to have a Major Accident Procedure which is flexible enough to deal with any type of accident. Whilst a hospital in a particular locality might expect a certain type of major accident due to the local industry, etc., it is now apparent in the light of experience in the last few years, for example, the Brighton Bombing and the Bradford City Fire, that a major receiving hospital must be prepared to meet any emergency and that no major accident plan can take every eventuality into account.

In summary the major lessons learned which are now being incorporated into a review of the Bradford procedure are:

Improved communications not only within the hospital, but also with other emergency services using modern communication technology;
A complete review of the cascade system of alerting staff (for example, instead of one person at the hospital telephoning all the members of staff needed to come in, he or she telephones one person, who in turn telephones another person before they set off, and so on), and the introduction of individual actions cards;
The permanent relocation of the control centre to an area immediately adjacent to the A&E department where the monitoring of activity can be more easily achieved and closer liaison with the police control centre;
Improved staff identification: difficulties were experienced by cer-

tain people because there were staff in civilian clothes;
Better communications with adjacent hospitals who may be required to take casualties and/or transfers of existing patients;
Information control must be set up jointly by the police and by administration;
It is vital that an area be set up away from clinical areas where arrangements for coping with the demand from distressed relatives can be carefully planned to ensure that information is given as effectively as possible, while avoiding serious interference with the hospital's primary tasks of caring for the casualties. Having said that, it must not be forgotten that these people are extremely worried for their loved ones and need constant support and reassurance; perhaps this is where social workers and clergy can be very useful. All information must be frequently updated;
Last, but certainly not least of the lessons to be learned, is that it is patently obvious that the only way of dealing with any major disaster is an effective triage system.

Control of press

It has long been recognised that intense media interest could pose enormous problems for hospitals during a major accident! Problems quite beyond the bounds of their everyday experience.

The clamour for information from relatives, press, television and radio may be the biggest single administration problem of a major accident. The underlying accuracy of this forecast was amply borne out at Bradford where, within 24 hours of the fire starting, a press corps approaching 100 had assembled in the city representing not just Britain's but the world's media. Calls were soon being received from both sides of the Atlantic, and there was intense interest from as far as Australia and New Zealand.

Within an hour of the fire, public relations officers from the Yorkshire Regional Health Authority had been drawn in to support local administration and to bear the brunt of media activity. Their support was maintained round the clock in the early stages of the disaster and continued on a daily basis until the last patient had been discharged.

The public relations officers did their job so effectively that on the afternoon and evening of the disaster neither my staff nor myself were aware of the presence of the media; we were completely protected. However, it was essential to add to the media's understanding of the situation so formal, controlled opportunities were set up to enable them to meet those intimately involved in the disaster, e.g., patients, doctors, nurses, administration and so on.

A regular programme of briefings, press conferences and visits was instituted from the outset to supplement the twice-daily bulletins on patients' conditions.

Press activity heightened with visits to the Bradford Royal Infirmary from the Prime Minister and the Health Minister which received widespread but lightly controlled media attention.

Because of the scale of facilities offered to the media, both reporters and photographers, there was no attempt by them to infiltrate hospitals wearing white coats, posing as National Health Service staff, as has been experienced elsewhere in similar situations.

Whether the Bradford fire taught us any new lessons in handling the media is perhaps questionable. However, it reinforced a number of already held beliefs and, certainly, the earliest possible involvement of the National Health Service's professional public relations officers is invaluable.

Conclusion

Whilst a number of things went wrong on the afternoon of 11 May a large number of things were right.

A normal Saturday afternoon in an A&E department was transformed in a matter of minutes into having to deal with one of the worst major accidents this century has ever witnessed. The fact that over 200 casualties were dealt with in a period of under four hours reflects the expertise and professionalism of staff in all disciplines within the hospital and, indeed, all the services involved.

As far as the staff at Bradford Royal Infirmary were concerned, to a large extent they mobilised themselves and each knew the role they had to play.

13

The Abbeystead Pumping Station explosion, 1984

Veronica Pickles and Stuart Westbrook

Introduction

The Abbeystead disaster proved that any disaster concerning the loss of life or severe injury is horrendous.

The disaster within itself was unique.

Royal Lancaster Infirmary

The Royal Lancaster Infirmary is the Acute General Hospital situated in the City of Lancaster and forms part of the Lancaster Health District. There are some 361 acute beds on the Infirmary site.

All major physical emergencies are admitted to this hospital and the ICU and Coronary Care Units (CCU) are also situated there.

The normal catchment area for the Infirmary extends north into Cumbria, as far as Tebay, south into Lancashire, as far as Preesall/Knott-End-on-Sea, and east into the Yorkshire Dales.

Abbeystead Pumping Station

On the evening of 23 May 1984, a group of approximately 40 people, mostly families, were visiting an underground pumping station at Abbeystead on the invitation of the North West Water Authority. All of these people were from the local village of St Michael and had suffered in past years from the effects of flooding when the nearby River Wyre had broken its banks after heavy rain. The tour of the Pumping Station was designed to explain its function and alleviate the fears of local people. During that e ning, all of them were caught in an underground explosion. An e: rmous fireball ripped through the station and tore a massive hole in the roof. Above ground, cars parked nearby were severely damaged by the blast. A car bonnet was later found several hundred metres from the vehicle. The sound of the blast was heard some kilometres away and local people raised the alarm and raced to the scene to give what assistance they could.

The Abbeystead Pumping Station is situated 10.5 km (6.5 miles) south west of Lancaster in the Trough of Bowland (see Fig. 13.1). This pleasant rural area is situated on the Duke of Westminster's Estate. The road access to the site is via mainly '3' class roads, and travelling time to the disaster scene was hampered due to the undulating geographical area.

Alert

At 19.50 hours, the A&E department at the Royal Lancaster Infirmary received a message from ambulance control warning of an explosion nearby and the possibility of numerous casualties. On duty were two trained and two untrained staff. The department itself had been unusually quiet that evening; the senior nurse immediately informed the clinical nurse manager on duty of the warning message and staff were placed on stand-by. Two or three minutes later this warning was upgraded to major accident with the possibility of approximately 30 to 40 casualties with severe burns. The time was 19.58 hours.

The Major Accident Procedure was put into action. All wards and departments and all duty doctors and consultants and other staff were alerted. Consultants went to their various wards to transfer patients or discharge those who could be discharged. It was visiting time, so most patients had transport available to them without stretching the ambulance service. It was nearly staff changeover time so fortunately nurses were availble to all areas of the hospital. Other staff, medical, nursing and non-nursing, all returned voluntarily to the hospital on hearing the news. Junior nursing staff from the nurses' home were brought across to assist. The duty clinical nurse manager took initial control and coordination of the disaster plan both quickly and efficiently.

The Abbeystead Pumping Station explosion, 1984

Mobile team

In the A&E department a team assembled to take the emergency equipment and medical staff to the scene, but there was no ambulance available. Our emergency equipment for a major accident is quite extensive and the police had only one unmarked vehicle available to transport both staff and equipment, so staff chose to use their own vehicles.

First casualties

The first casualties were arriving at the A&E department by 20.05 hours. Three people were helped out of a car driven by one of the locals who had been first on the scene. It was apparent that they were suffering from severe burns. Their hair was badly singed and most of their clothing was burned off. They were distressed, in severe pain, and shocked. Extra medical staff were available and, as casualties arrived, they were delegated to various areas by the coordinating nurse. They received basic resuscitation and treatment and were reassured. They were then admitted to the wards for further treatment and dressings.

Medical and surgical supplies

Medical and surgical supplies between ward and department areas need to be constantly reviewed so that overstocking of some items and understocking of others is carefully monitored and corrected. The Infirmary is fortunate in having its own district medical and surgical supplies close by and was not hampered by having a centralised store system. The sterile supply stocks were depleting quickly and extras were sent for urgently. Pharmacy held a civil stock of Diamorphine which was counted out on arrival at casualty and counted back after all the casualties had left the department. The coordinating nurse had responsibility for this.

Human plasma protein fraction stocks were soon exhausted and plasma expanders were used as a substitute. Stocks of Flamazine which were used for most of the dressings were also soon depleted.

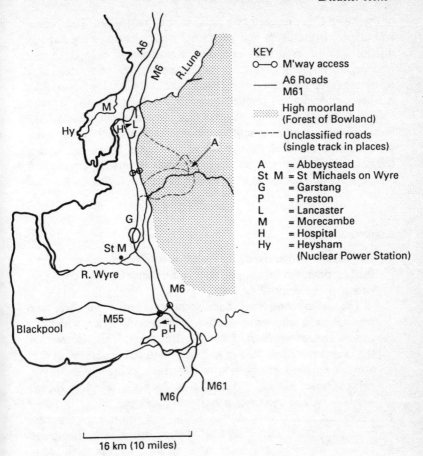

KEY
○—○ M'way access
———— A6 Roads
     M61
∷∷∷ High moorland
     (Forest of Bowland)
- - - - Unclassified roads
     (single track in places)

A   = Abbeystead
St M = St Michaels on Wyre
G   = Garstang
P   = Preston
L   = Lancaster
M   = Morecambe
H   = Hospital
Hy   = Heysham
     (Nuclear Power Station)

16 km (10 miles)

Fig. 13.1 Abbeystead and surrounding area.

Disaster scene

As the mobile team arrived at the scene, it was discovered that the majority of the casualties had already been transported back to the Royal Lancaster Infirmary; some went to Preston Royal Infirmary direct, but the team remained on stand-by in case of any more survivors. It was not known at this point just how many people had been inside the station when the accident happened or in fact, how many had been rescued. Fire and ambulance personnel had, at risk of their own lives, rescued two badly injured casualties. The police, ambulance, fire officers and personnel were working very hard in difficult conditions at the scene. The explosion had caused the roof to collapse, trapping casualties and hampering rescue work. There was danger of the roof collapsing further, together with rubble, further hampering the rescue operation. Looking into the massive hole in the ground, it was obvious that some had not survived the blast. These casualties could have been certified at the scene, but were transported back to the Royal Lancaster Infirmary, and a temporary mortuary was set up in the outpatients department. A senior nurse and doctor were delegated to receive them.

Communications

1 As patients had arrived, they were identified by numbers until further details were sought after admission. Clerical staff gave details to the controlling team.

   The team comprised administrative, senior nursing, and medical staff, who set up control in the general office, which is a central area of the Royal Lancaster Infirmary. This also became the communications centre and dealt with all problems as they arose, i.e., the identification of casualties, contacting relatives, press release, beddage, condition of patients, laundry, theatre availability, and catering for staff and relatives.

2 Communications between the disaster site and the hospital base is of paramount importance. However, this may be hampered through sheer geographical environment, and an early communication network is essential to relay messages from the site to the receiving hospital. These messages should be short, precise and clear, and coordination between other emergency services is obviously of the greatest importance.

3 The network of information from the site to the department and from the department to wards through the central control is vital.

4 As happened in the Abbeystead disaster, the speed of the incident could have led to information being incorrect or going astray, or not reaching all relevant parties. It is therefore essential that all paperwork and documentation is kept as normal and no special data is produced for specific use in a major disaster. Flow charts in the department and in central control have now been

developed and colour coding is used for the patient's name as to their triage condition.

The coordinating nurse in the department is very important. The role should initially be adopted by the most senior nurse on duty in the department, with more senior personnel relieving as required.

5 Action cards have been developed for use by the senior nurse in charge of the department following this disaster and are reviewed and updated as necessary.

6 Ward and department status sheets have also been developed. Therefore, when a disaster is declared, the senior officer on duty can instruct all wards to complete their ward status forms and will very quickly and easily have documented status of each ward and department with regard to the number of patients ready for discharge, transfer, laundry, CSSD, pharmacy, etc. Wards that can then be used for initial transfer or admission of patients are identified very easily.

Switchboard

It is essential that switchboard draft additional operators in as soon as possible. Workload through the switchboard becomes very demanding. Enquiries, referrals, etc., can soon block the board. As a result of this disaster, the requesting of a second switchboard operative, or more, becomes a high priority on the recall list.

Press

There must be a central control and information centre for the press and relatives. Regular information and press releases must be given to the press and only by doing this can one ensure that the correct information is being sent out.

Casualty admissions complete

By 21.30 hours all the casualties had been admitted to a ward, to the operating theatre, or to the ICU. The department was cleared and reopened in one to one and a half hours. Staff left the department around midnight. In total, 44 patients came to the casualty department, the majority suffering from 60% to 80% burns and a few with the complication of trauma. Two patients were admitted to the ICU. Eight people went direct to the Preston Royal Infirmary from the scene. The majority of these eight were also suffering from trauma. One man had miraculously suffered only minor burns to his hands and was later discharged. Over the next few weeks there were to be more deaths, and it was very distressing when one realised that husbands, wives, sons and daughters all from the same community were tragically separated in this terrible accident.

Teamwork

The importance of teamwork cannot be stressed enough. It was very pleasing to see the hospital team swing into action. Domestic staff returned to the hospital where they did a sterling job of clearing the department and wards ready for the next admission. Portering, catering, pharmacy, pathology, laundry, CSSD, and many many other staff, provided the department and the ward areas with a service that was second to none.

Counselling service

What is important is the need for a counselling service to all members of staff involved in any disaster (see Chapter 7). Provision of such a counselling service proved to be very successful with learner nurses and would have served to be very advantageous if extended to all members of staff involved.

Equipment

The major disaster equipment within the department had fortunately only recently been reviewed before the Abbeystead disaster and therefore no radical changes were made, apart from removing blood crossmatch bottles, etc., from the disaster kit. While it may be advantageous for blood samples to be made prior to the patient's transfer to the receiving centre, the risk of error at the site far outweighs any advantage. Difficulties with transportation of the disaster team, plus its equipment, have been resolved by the purchase of a purpose-built Flying Squad Emergency Vehicle. This has been made available through public donations. Provision of Accidental Injury Insurance to members of the Flying Squad/Major Accident Team has been reviewed and arrangements have been made for personal accident insurance.

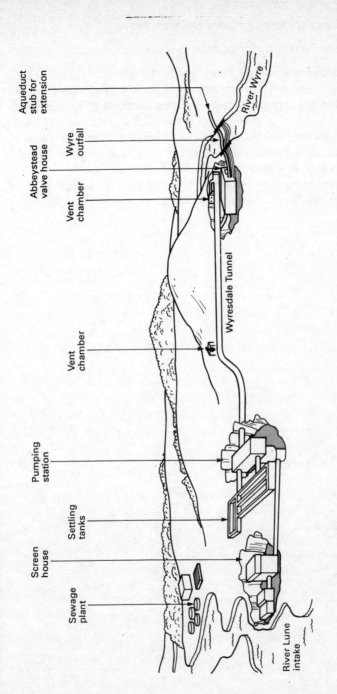

Fig. 13.2 Overall layout of the Lune – Wyre transfer scheme.

The Abbeystead Pumping Station explosion, 1984

Stability and efficiency throughout the disaster

We are very fortunate in Lancaster to have experienced medical staff who maintained stability throughout the disaster, and whose instructions were clear, precise, and a common understanding was therefore achieved by all. Nursing staff in the A&E department and wards are professional, and extremely capable people. They coped admirably with this disaster and adapted with ease to the increased demands that were made upon them.

All the emergency services involved displayed a high level of efficiency and they liaised closely and professionally throughout.

14

A motorway crash: the M6 disaster, 1985

Michael McColl

The accident took place on the southbound carriageway of the M6 Motorway just north of Preston, Lancashire (see Fig. 14.1), one beautiful October day in 1985. Traffic was being compressed into a single lane on account of routine road repairs, and had come to a standstill because of the congestion. A Glasgow to London express coach, carrying 42 passengers, failed to slow down and crashed at speed into a car containing two adults. The car was pushed into three others before bursting into flames, with its two occupants trapped inside. The coach ploughed on, striking and mounting two further cars which each contained two adults and two children; all were killed on impact. Petrol from the ruptured tanks ignited as all three vehicles slid along the motorway, and flames were sucked in through the shattered windscreen of the coach. The burning mass then struck a van which in turn hit another car; these both caught fire. Several other knock-on collisions then took place; 13 vehicles in all were involved. Coach passengers strugged to the rear exit as flames spread rapidly through the bus. Those hesitating at the four foot drop were unceremoniously pushed out. Motorists immediately behind the crash left their cars to assist the injured lying on the motorway.

At 13.24 hours Hutton Police Headquarters, South Preston, received a call from a member of the public on the motorway. There had been a bad accident on the M6 southbound carriageway; people were trapped, cars were on fire and the carriageway was blocked. Four police patrol cars were directed to the incident, and ambulance and fire services were notified. Police arrived on the scene two minutes later and were confronted by a shambolic landscape of battered vehicles spread across the motorway, some of which were burning furiously. Southbound traffic was piling up by the minute.

A motorway crash: the M6 disaster, 1985

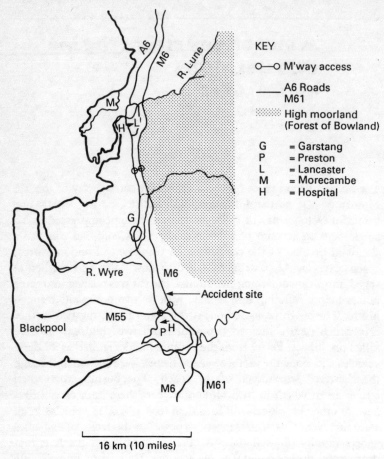

Fig. 14.1 Map indicating site of accident and location of hospital.

A pillar of smoke marked the scene. The Preston Fire Engine struggled through northbound motorway traffic which had slowed in curious horror; at times a runner was used to disperse obstructing cars and a crossover point was anxiously searched for – fortunately one was found at the accident site! A fire engine from Garstang, north of the accident, raced south along the hard shoulder.

Senior ambulance officers arrived, took stock of the situation, and began triaging the injured. The police had meanwhile closed the motorway, north and south, at Junctions 32 and 33. The lower closure was complicated by the M55 joining it. Firemen, having established that no lives could be saved in the fire, began hosing the flames with water and foam. Colleagues found a water source $1\frac{1}{2}$ km (1 mile) away – too far for the hoses, so water was carried to the accident site in a fire engine. Two gas cylinders were found, hosed and identified, and gently placed in a makeshift water-filled trough to prevent an explosion. Ambulances began ferrying the more seriously injured to hospital. Passengers from the coach and involved cars who had escaped unhurt, or relatively so, had crossed the northbound carriageway and waited or wandered on the grass embankment beyond the hard shoulder. They were joined by a large number of spectators. Ambulancemen had difficulty sorting out these people and found it easier to label those who did not require attention rather than those who did. The down-draught from the helicopters which were hovering overhead was fanning the flames of burning vehicles and blowing blankets, papers, etc., around the site. The police had to wave them away before they could begin the job of turning round the southbound carriageway traffic jam, now several kilometres long, and sending the vehicles north up the southbound carriageway and off at Junction 33.

As firemen struggled to extinguish the motorway fire, patients were arriving at the Royal Preston Hospital A&E Department. Major accident experience had been obtained in the Abbeystead disaster; staff waited, anxious but confident. A control group, comprising a senior doctor, senior nurse and senior hospital administrator run the hospital, whilst the accident controller manages the casualty department, advising and making requests of the main control group as necessary. The hospital has 900 beds; most specialities including those of plastic surgery and neurosurgery are on site. A&E department policy is to try to provide a casualty officer for every seriously injured patient. The casualty officer takes full charge of the patient, enlisting help and advice, and supervising moves to the X-ray department or elsewhere. He/she informs the control group of the patient's diagnosis, whereabouts and progress. Specialist advice is immediately available. Minor injuries are attended to in an adjacent area.

In total, 38 people were brought to the A&E department; and 27 required attention. Of the 27, 15 had only minor injuries and were discharged after treatment. In the end, 12 patients were admitted with a number of injuries, including a wedged thoracic vertebra, a hip dislocation, three head injuries and two with burns to the face and hands, one of whom was admitted to the ICU. Several of these people also suffered from the effects of smoke inhalation.

It is not satisfactory to have patients linger unnecessarily within the department, and all of them were either discharged or admitted within the hour. Those people who had been brought in from the accident unhurt were comforted and catered for in a separate area. Most of those admitted were discharged within a day or so; only two were kept longer than two weeks.

At the accident site forensic photographs were taken. Three bodies had been found in the burnt out coach. The full extent of the tragedy became apparent as firemen released charred bodies from their unyielding metal envelopes – all that remained of the two cars under the coach front. The bodies were wrapped in plastic bags and transferred to the mortuary of another Preston hospital; identification took several days. Uninjured coach passengers had been taken to a local hotel. Preston police contacted the coach owners who arranged transport for those wishing to continue their journey, and they also liaised with police north of the Lancashire border who contacted relatives of the injured patients and, subsequently, the relatives of those who had died. Both the hospital and police headquarters were swamped by the huge number of enquiries about the incident.

A meeting was later held to discuss problems that had arisen in the major accident. On the hospital side, previous experience indicated that the hospital control group should remain in the A&E department with the accident controller; this worked well. The police had been unhappy about the location of their incident room and had moved to an office adjoining the A&E department. The ambulance service was concerned that the hospital closed its doors to other ambulance cases during the incident and four patients were diverted elsewhere. Retrospectively, though this was a part of the Major Accident Plan, further pressure was put on the ambulance service and a small number of people inconvenienced. In future, hospital and ambulance controls will discuss diversions before taking any action. (Outpatient clinics had carried on normally throughout the afternoon.)

It was noted that no medical emergency team had been called out, though the local general practitioners run an immediate care scheme. There is also an arrangement where a number of interested GPs would be prepared to work on site if requested to do so; the A&E department also runs an ambulance-based flying squad. It was not felt that any of the patients would have benefitted significantly from on site medical care. Moreover, the accident occurred very near the hospital and patients were transferred within a few minutes. Some of the hospital's departments were felt to have been sluggish in implementing their part of the Major Accident Plan, and the workload for the clerical staff was felt to have been underestimated.

The M6 motorway disaster was the worst in English motorway history. In total 13 vehicles were involved, 13 people died, 27 required hospital attention, and half of these were admitted. Both northbound and southbound carriageways of the motorway were closed for several hours. Though the accident was eventually attributed to driver error, a number of problems were highlighted. Express coaches had to travel at speeds in excess of 110 k.p.h. (70 m.p.h.) to maintain their schedules. The motorway lane adjustments and closures had all been properly indicated, but the quality of the signposting was queried, and the danger of leaving only a single lane open was discussed. All the vehicles involved in the accident were carefully examined, in particular the coach which had caught fire and become a wind tunnel of flames within the space of two to three minutes. It was not until a further disastrous accident occurred on the M61 motorway, in which another 13 people were killed, that vigorous action was taken (to a considerable extent because of local press publicity) and speeding restrictions at motorway repairs firmly enforced.

The most dangerous motorway hazard is a stationary vehicle or a group of them.

15

Nuclear disaster planning after Chernobyl, 1986

The last ten years have introduced the world to the possibility of a major nuclear accident. Chernobyl in the Soviet Union and Three Mile Island (TMI) in the United States have made us all aware of the potential for disaster inherent in the nuclear industry. However, this needs to be considered in perspective for 'conventional' industry can be extremely hazardous as well. Large scale operations, for example, mining, have been responsible for accidents with death tolls in the hundreds, while the chemical industry has the potential to contaminate extensive areas with leakages of highly toxic gases such as happened tragically at Bophal in India.

The purpose of this chapter is therefore to consider any accidents that may have happened in the UK, before describing TMI and Chernobyl. It concludes with a discussion of the current state of planning in the UK to cope with a nuclear accident at a British power station.

The safety record of the British nuclear industry is extremely good, with the one possible exception of the plant operated by British Nuclear Fuels Limited (BNFL) at Sellafield, formerly Windscale, in Cumbria. A serious accident occurred in October 1957 involving the nuclear reactor that is on the site (Dace, 1987). The temperature rose to fuel melting point as a result of operator error; the readings on temperature gauges related to a cooler part of the core, not the problem section as thought at the time. It took 42 hours before the problem was correctly diagnosed, and by this time there was a fire involving the graphite moderator in the core (this 'moderates' the energy of the neutrons in order to aid the nuclear reactions going on in the core and the uranium fuel). The fire was put out on 11 October by flooding the core with large quantities of water, risking an explosion in the process. Fortunately this worked and the fire was put out. Various calculations concerning the amount of radioactivity released suggested that some 260 cases of cancer would be caused, of which 33 would be fatal. Vast quantities of milk were thrown away over an area of 500 square kilometres (193 square miles) in the aftermath.

What is particularly disturbing is that the public were told nothing until 24 hours after the fire had started and were then told that the radioactive material had blown out to sea when it had blown inland. The National Radiological Protection Board (NRPB) report into the incident was not published until 1983, a delay of 26 years (Dace, 1987).

The early 1980s saw a series of embarrassing accidents and leaks also occurring at Sellafield which led to major public concern over the safety of the plant, especially in the aftermath of the TMI incident. Fortunately the management have acted to improve standards at the plant, and to improve public access to information about the nuclear industry, a move paralleled by the CEGB. It would be totally unforgiveable if the public were ever deceived in the same way as they were in 1957.

The range of possible nuclear accidents and the sort of response that would be needed by the emergency services in the UK is considered below. Chernobyl and TMI are clearly uppermost in most people's minds when considering nuclear accidents, so these two situations shall be discussed first.

Three Mile Island

The TMI incident began on Wednesday 28 March 1979 when a series of plant failures were compounded by operator errors. A site emergency was declared at 07.00 hours when all nonessential personnel were sent home. The news media began carrying the story at 10.00 hours. The problem arose because part of the reactor cooling system had been accidentally shut down and the back up system failed to operate due to incorrect closure of key valves at an earlier stage. Further valve malfunction led to the loss of thousands of gallons of cooling water which in turn led to the automatic switching on of emergency cooling pumps. Unfortunately, human error intervened again as the operators misjudged the situation and shut off the vital emergency cooling pumps. The result was overheating and core damage leading to a radioactive release and a collection of hydrogen gas within the core that threatened a major explosion.

On Friday 30 March 1979, Governor Richard Thornburg urged pregnant women and children under the age of five living within eight km (five miles) of the plant to leave the area. A total of 23 schools within this area were closed. Dace (1987) has commented on the disruption to families that occurred in this stage of the evacuation, resulting in children being separated from their parents. Residents within 16 km (10 miles) of the plant were being urged to stay indoors and keep doors and windows closed while plans were being formulated for the mass evacuation of 950 000 people within a 32 km (20 mile) radius of TMI. Radiation levels in the vicinity of the plant were now reading 0.8 mSv per hour (Lesher and Bomberger, 1979). For comparison, this level almost equals the maximum permitted *annual* dose, from artificial sources (1 mSv), for the general public in the UK.

Lesher and Bomberger (1979) have described how large numbers of people were leaving the area, even though there were as yet no major evacuation requirements. It is significant that these authors, both senior nurses at the Lebanon County Hospital, describe their own feelings of uncertainty and lack of understanding of what was happening. By Sunday 1 April it was estimated that 200 000 people had left the area and curfews had been imposed, indicating large scale distrust of the authorities by the population. Staffing problems had become acute at surrounding hospitals as staff simply left the area, regardless of duty requirements. It is easy to see major problems for the police trying to control this exodus, and also the potential for looting and theft due to the large number of empty homes and shops left behind.

A major aggravating factor of the TMI incident was the handling of news and information. The pressure from the media for news interfered with the functioning of the incident management team and at times incorrect information was broadcast. Breo (1979) has reported the result of a mistaken broadcast which was to the effect that a large release of xenon gas has occurred on Friday 30 March. The outcome was that the switchboard of the Herschey Medical Center, a 300 bed acute hospital 12.5 km (8 miles) from TMI, was jammed for 10 hours with hysterical callers. Clearly this severely interferes with the hospital's functioning. Among those unable to get through on the telephone that day was the hospital's Emergency Director, Dr Muller, who was at a meeting in San Francisco. Breo has described that when the hospital was warned on 31 March of the possibility of the ultimate risk, a meltdown or explosion due to the hydrogen bubble referred to earlier, it was decided that evacuation was likely. The hospital managed to discharge 200 patients in 48 hours. Breo recalls how many of the patients did not need much persuasion to go home! Plans for evacuation to hospitals well out of the area were coordinated at State level, and the Herschey Center was ready to transfer its remaining 100 patients via ambulances and trucks to wherever indicated. Most hospitals in the area were able to discharge about 50% of their patients within 48 hours, and had similar plans ready. It is interesting to speculate how long it would take the average UK general hospital to discharge 50% of its patients in a similar situation.

Fortunately the first few days of April saw the situation under control and the reactor eventually safely shut down. The major effects on people were stress related with relatively small radiation releases.

Could a TMI scenario develop in the UK? The reactor at TMI is completely different from any in use in the UK, depending as it did upon water to act as a coolant (PWR); UK reactors use carbon dioxide gas for this function. Older reactors are known as Magnox Reactors after the fuel rod system they use, and modern reactors are called AGRs, Advanced Gas Cooled Reactors. Given the different nature of the reactors, the CEGB are confident that TMI could not happen at any of the existing plants in the UK.

The next generation of nuclear power stations in the UK will be built according to the American PWR system. However, since TMI, many lessons have been learnt and substantial extra safety features built into the PWR system.

The striking feature of the TMI incident is the way humans behaved, both in terms of individual operator error and collectively as a population around the site. The reader is referred to Chapter 7 for a fuller discussion of the psychology involved in disasters.

Chernobyl

Seven years after TMI, the world's worst nuclear accident occurred at Chernobyl in the Ukraine. At 01.23 hours local time, 26 April 1986, number four reactor exploded. The disaster occurred in the process of an experiment being carried out as the reactor was being shut down for maintenance. It is worth stressing that nuclear reactors cannot explode in the same way as a nuclear bomb; the way they are constructed makes this impossible.

However, a 'conventional' explosion is possible and in the case of Chernobyl two actually happened. The first explosion blew off the 1000 tonne concrete upper neutron shield, and the second wrecked the large reactor building.

The sequence of events at Chernobyl has been well described by Gittus (1987) who has shown how the disaster had its origins in a mixture of bad reactor design and human error. Without going into the detailed physics of the situation, a major problem with the Chernobyl RBMK reactor was that it was unstable if operated at less than 20% of full power. Unfortunately, there was nothing to prevent the operator running the reactor at less than 20% full power except instructions to this effect. No automatic safety systems existed to shut the reactor down if this was attempted.

A further problem with the RBMK reactor was the slowness of the manually operated emergency shut down system. All reactors have a system of control rods which can be introduced or removed from the reactor, the purpose of which is to absorb and control the flow of neutrons within the reactor. This neutron flow controls the rate of nuclear reactions and hence heat generation.

The scene was then set for disaster as the operator began an unauthorised experiment, operating the reactor at a power level that was expressly forbidden. Within seconds the temperature of the core began to rise as the instability of the reactor began a process of positive feedback. The operator pressed the emergency shut down button, but the system was too slow to deal with the situation. A power surge took place leading to the sudden production of large quantities of steam within the core and also the melting and disintegration of the fuel. It was this steam that caused the first explosion. The reaction of the steam and zirconium alloy tubes that run through the core (88 mm (3.25 inches) outside diameter, walls 4 mm (0.25 inches) thick; function, to carry the fuel assemblies) produced hydrogen, that in turn reacted with air in the reactor hall to produce the second explosion. This explosion wrecked the building and threw solid pieces of radioactive fuel over the surrounding area.

Some 30 fires were started in the vicinity as pieces of burning radioactive core material fell to ground. The core was now exposed to the atmosphere and the graphite moderator (graphite is carbon, as in charcoal) caught fire. Large amounts of radioactive material were thus able to escape into the atmosphere, assisted by the thermal effects of the blazing core. Ironically, this probably reduced the radiation casualty toll in the immediate area as the highly radioactive material was rapidly lifted high into the atmosphere, reducing radiation levels close by the plant to less than they might have been.

The initial explosion led to two deaths and within 25 minutes the first casualties were being treated at Pripyat Hospital, 4 km (2.5 miles) away. The Soviet authorities staged a massive response to the disaster and within hours had flown to the scene the first of 230 medical teams consisting of doctors, nurses and technicians. In the first 24 hours they had seen and treated some 1000 people.

The initial criteria used for treating radiation casualties were; time since vomiting began, gastrointestinal symptoms and skin condition, along with white cell counts. Reference to p. 44 shows the significance of these parameters in estimating radiation exposure.

It is estimated that 200 people had received doses of over 1 gray (Gy) (approximately equivalent to 1 Sv, see Table 3.5), 50 of whom had received over 5 Gy. Doses were of either external gamma or beta radiation, and by inhalation of gaseous fission products. On 27 April, the most severely affected patients (129 in total) were airlifted to Moscow for specialist treatment at the Moscow Hospital Number 6. The following day saw another 170 patients airlifted to Moscow.

Most of the worst casualties were among station staff and rescue and fire fighting teams. There were undoubtedly many acts of heroism performed in the aftermath of the explosion, and many staff fought the fires knowing they were exposing themselves to probably fatal doses of radiation. The slow death of radiation sickness had claimed seven victims by 15 May, and the death toll stood at 31 by October 1986 despite the most intensive and sophisticated medical efforts, including 19 bone marrow transplants.

The authorities began dumping large amounts of solid material, totalling some 5000 tonnes, on the core to reduce the release of radioactive materials. While this had the desired effect for the first few days, it also had the effect of providing the core with thermal insulation leading to an increase in temperature. By 4–5 May the core temperature underneath the mound of solid material had risen to 190°C and radioactive release was increasing again in response to the increased temperature. The Soviet authorities then began a programme of nitrogen injection underneath the core to prevent oxygen reaching the core, thereby preventing combustion. The nitrogen also acted as a coolant and brought the situation under control, establishing a stable temperature with minimal radioactivity release. Chernobyl Number 4 reactor has since been effectively entombed.

The evacuation that followed cleared the town of Pripyat of its 45 000 population in three hours with the help of 1100 buses. Over the weekend of 3 and 4 May, the evacuation zone was extended out to a 30 km (19 miles) radius requiring the relocation of 100 000 people, all of whom were examined for radiation effects by a team of 5000 medical staff. The final evacuation total stood at 135 000, plus hundreds of thousands of farm animals.

Nuclear accidents and the UK

The CEGB are quite right to point out that an accident similar to Chernobyl could not happen in the UK as reactors of that type do not exist here and, further, if such a design had been proposed, it would never have been licensed because of its poor safety features. Consideration of Chernobyl and TMI however leave a series of questions to be answered. What are the risks and scenarios for a UK nuclear accident? What has happened after the Chernobyl explosion? What lessons can be learnt? Finally, what is the possibility of a nuclear accident elsewhere in Europe and how might that effect the UK? These questions are addressed in the remainder of this chapter beginning with an analysis of nuclear risks in the UK.

Radioactive materials are in widespread use in industry, hospitals and research establishments, therefore accidents are possible. The concern, however, is for a major incident with the civilian nuclear power industry (CEGB and BNFL) and the military as the main areas for concern.

A civilian accident will not involve a nuclear explosion; the principle source of hazard to most people would be from exposure to radiation contained in a cloud of escaped material, mostly gaseous. To produce an explosive release of energy requires atoms of Uranium 235 or Plutonium 239 to be held together close enough and long enough for millions of atomic fission reactions to occur very rapidly. In a bomb this is achieved by explosive charges driving the fissile material together. It has already been stated that, unlike a nuclear warhead, a nuclear reactor cannot explode. A nuclear reactor contains mostly U238, diluting the small amount of U235 present. As the material is spread out in space to prevent it forming a compact enough mass, in the event of a core explosion, as happened at Chernobyl, the effect would be to blow the fissile material apart, rather than together as required in a bomb.

For these reasons, the possibility of a nuclear explosion from civilian scenarios can be eliminated. What then is the possibility of an accident at a UK power station resulting in the release of radioactive material into the environment? The answer is very remote indeed as the nuclear electricity generating industry has placed safety at the top of its list of priorities. It is probably fair to say that nuclear power stations are as safe as any piece of engineering can be, but is that safe enough?

Power station safety design

There are two steps necessary to produce a major environmental leak. Firstly, there has to be a malfunction within the system and, secondly, there has to be leakage of the fuel clad and a failure of the containment system to allow radioactivity out into the environment. In designing power stations engineers have consistently sought to identify potential malfunctions, and design plants in such a way as to eliminate or minimise the possibility of an environmental leak occurring, while at the same time building in safety precautions which can be activated in the event of a problem actually happening.

Reactors therefore have built-in redundancy, which in engineering terms means that there is more material available to do any job than is needed. If a failure occurs, there will always be enough material left to carry on functioning safely. As a simple analogy, it's like wearing a pair of braces and a belt to keep your trousers up. If the belt suddenly gives way, you still have your braces to spare any blushes! Features such as this and multiple fail-safe systems designed to shut the reactor down automatically when something does not happen, rather than having to wait for something to happen, all combine to maximise safety.

The second component of reactor safety involves containment systems. Radioactive fuel is contained in stainless steel tubes which are contained within the graphite core which is in turn contained within a massive prestressed concrete pressure vessel over 4 metres (13 feet) thick, all of which is contained within a large reactor hall.

Engineers have spent a lot of time analysing all conceivable accidents in order to calculate the possible frequency of occurrence. A second analysis can then look at the possibility of a containment failure happening at the same time as a plant malfunction, the product of the two being an estimated probability of any given accident and its environmental implications.

An example of such an approach is given by Griffiths (1978) in a paper looking at Magnox and PWR accidents. This rigorous and technical analysis can be summarised by saying that if accidents likely to occur more than once in a million years are considered, the size of the area around a reactor where evacuation would be required is between 2–6 km (1.25–3.75 miles) in diameter depending on the type of reactor.

For this reason the CEGB do not consider accidents of greater severity worthy of serious planning as their probability of occurrence is less than once in a million years.

However, it is possible to consider the worst case scenarios such as a meltdown and, however remote the possibility, look at the effects that would have. Dace (1987) describes three studies of such a worst case scenario at the site of the proposed Dungeness PWR in Kent with a probability of 1 in 10 million per year. They found that assuming it was a day of gusty winds and rain, the population of Hythe, Dymchurch and Rye (total 30 000) could receive fatal doses of radiation, depending on wind direction, within a few days. Taking the worse case to its extreme, if the wind blew steadily from the south east it would carry a radioactive plume to London that would cause radiation-induced cancer deaths totalling 80 000, unless the whole population of London was evacuated for 20 years.

The problem facing planners and the emergency services relates to the balance between increasingly unlikely scenarios and the increasing amount of hazard each situation brings with it. Where can the line be drawn and it said that there is no point in planning beyond this point as the risk is so remote, however awful the consequences of an accident may be? It might be fair to say that the risk of a major, worst case scenario for a UK nuclear power station is about the same as a large meteorite striking the earth, an event which would have global consequences. There is no easy solution to this dilemma of where the planning cut-off point for disaster should be.

In considering the probability of a nuclear accident there are two non-technical causes: human error, which played a major role at Chernobyl and TMI; and also terrorism. UK reactors are designed to safeguard against operator error, as far as possible, with an extensive series of automatic safety systems all of which tend towards shutting the reactor down. Human error then is likely to shut the reactor down rather than cause an accident.

Terrorism is a possible threat. However, it would need a well-organised, well-armed group to take control of a nuclear power station. In such an eventuality, the reactor could be shut down by the simple step of isolating the station from the national grid. This could be easily done from outside the station, regardless of what was happening inside. Given the fail-safe systems built into the reactor, the CEGB are confident that, while it would be possible to cause a lot of damage to the reactor by deliberately operating the controls in such a way, it would not be possible to engineer a major environmental disaster, assuming action had not been taken to shut down the reactor.

As far as using explosives to attack the reactor, large amounts of sophisticated military explosives would be needed to blast through the many metres of concrete and steel that protect the core. It should be pointed out that there are access ports for various pipes through the concrete shielding which a demolitions expert might be able to breach, but this would still not expose the core. Any successful breaching of the core containment would put the terrorist at the same risk of death from escaping radioactivity as the surrounding population. It should also be remembered that a power station covers a vast area, unlike the closed confines of an aeroplane, which would make it very difficult for terrorists to ward off counter-terrorist actions by the security forces. However, vigilance and a high level of security against such possible operations are essential. Complacency, after all, recently allowed a young German pilot to fly his light aircraft through all the Soviet air defences and land in Red Square, Moscow!

CEGB plans

CEGB power stations have detailed plans drawn up to deal with accidents, and these are fully exercised every year. The minimum number of staff on duty at any one time is about 50, dispersed over a large area. The implications of this for an accident are that the emergency services are likely to have to cope with only a few 'conventional' casualties who may be contaminated or irradiated. The accident will only reach major proportions if it involves the release of radioactive material into the atmosphere.

It is worth noting the exact definitions used by the CEGB. A *site incident* involves a hazardous condition, the effects of which are expected to be confined within the site perimeter fence. An *emergency* however means that the situation is likely to cause a radiological hazard to the public in the vicinity of the station. These are two very different conditions, each of which can have alert and stand-by phases; stand-by indicating that the power station authorities believe there is an imminent risk of the full emergency situation developing.

The aims of a CEGB site emergency plan can be summarised as; safely accounting for all personnel on site, evacuating casualties to appropriate medical facilities, notifying the emergency services and taking whatever steps are needed to protect the population in the immediate vicinity. In addition, of course, power station staff will be seeking to bring the incident under control and terminate any hazard situation as quickly as possible.

One of the first authorities that the CEGB would contact in the event of an accident is the Meteorological Office to obtain accurate predictions about wind speed and direction, atmospheric turbulence, rainfall, etc., all of which are essential elements in predicting downwind radiation levels. Staff from the emergency services should be guided by CEGB personnel at all times as the CEGB will be operating a monitoring system that will indicate radiation levels. Radiation acts on the human body in a cumulative way, i.e., twice the dose, twice the risk. Time exposed to radiation is therefore crucial; a ten minute exposure is twice as hazardous as a five minute exposure for any level of radiation.

In the early stages of the emergency the site personnel monitor radation levels and deal with the cause of the problem, possibly with support from the fire brigade, while the ambulance service evacuate any injured persons to hospital. Priority for evacuation depends on clinical condition not contamination levels. If there is time to decontaminate a casualty at the power station, then that is permissable. However, if their condition does not permit this, they should be moved, in accordance with the agreed protocol for contaminated casualties, to the correct A&E unit immediately for resuscitation and treatment. Such an agreed protocol exists for all nuclear power stations with local hospital A&E units, and it should be well known to all parties and regularly practised, otherwise it is not worth the paper it is written on.

Chernobyl brought the use of iodine blocking tablets to many people's attention. A likely component of any release from a reactor is a radioactive isotope of iodine. Iodine is concentrated and stored in the thyroid gland of man, therefore it is possible that the radioactive form would be sufficiently concentrated in the gland to give rise to cancer of the thyroid. This has long been recognised as possible, and the recommended preventative measure has been to take a stable type of iodine in the form of a tablet; the effect of which is to fill all the potential storage sites in the thyroid with non-radioactive iodine. If a person were then to inhale the radioactive form, the gland could not concentrate the isotope in the thyroid as there would be no sites available to store it, thereby greatly reducing the risk of developing cancer of the thyroid in later life.

Iodine tablets only protect against cancer of the thyroid, and to be fully effective they should ideally be taken *before* the person inhales substantial amounts of radioactive iodine. There are large stocks of iodine tablets, running into thousands, held jointly by the CEGB at their plants and by police forces in the area; the exact number varying with the population in the vicinity of the plant. Iodine tablets are therefore an essential *early* requirement of any local plan, particularly for CEGB personnel and rescue workers.

As an incident unfolds, the CEGB will set up an Operation Support Centre (OSC). This concept has its origins amongst the lessons learnt from TMI where it was felt effective management of the emergency site was not possible because of media pressure and the demands made for information from a whole range of State and Federal bodies. The OSC is envisaged as a fully equipped control centre which will deal with the media, provide information for the emergency services, the EPO team (Chapter 6), and local and other authorities, and generally act as a coordinating focal point for the whole operation. This will leave the control centre at the power station free to get on with the job of dealing with the actual site problem. It is envisaged that within hours of an incident commencing a Government Technical Advisor (GTA) will be present at the OSC to take charge of operations.

Decisions about evacuation will be based upon what are known as Emergency Reference Levels (ERL) which were originally drawn up by the National Radiological Protection Board (NRPB) as criteria for limiting doses of radiation to the public in the event of an accident. The NRPB envisages that these levels would be used as the basis for planning evacuation and other measures in the first 12 hours or so after an incident (NRPB, 1981).

An ERL is given as a range of values. The NRPB consider that below the lower level, the risk from countermeasures is greater than the risk from radiation. However, when the lower level is reached, consideration should be given to countermeasures, and when the upper limit is reached, the NRPB regards countermeasures as mandatory whatever the circumstances. Table 15.1 summarises the current ERLs.

Table 15.1 Current emergency reference levels (ERL).

Countermeasure	Whole body dose range	
	Lower ERL	Upper ERL
Evacuation	100 mSv	500 mSv
Shelter indoors	5 mSv	25 mSv

It is possible to calculate doses for different organs. For example, the ERLs for the thyroid gland are 50–250 mSv where the counter-measure of giving stable iodine is concerned. The NRPB calculates that a whole body dose of 100 mSv carries with it a 1:1000 risk of death due to radiation effects (cancer).

The cumulative effect of radiation should be remembered here, thus an accident that produced contamination at the rate of 20 mSv per hour would need five hours to give the downwind population a sufficient dose that evacuation should be considered, ERL 100 mSv. The nearest large town to Chernobyl is Pripyat. This was evacuated when, 24 hours later, radiation levels had reached approximately 5 mSv per hour. Therefore, there is unlikely to be a need for an instant evacuation, and things can proceed in an orderly manner over a period of hours or even a day or two. Panic must be avoided at all costs as not only does this pose extra hazards to evacuees, it also impairs the ability of the emergency services to deal with the situation.

Reference has been made to the fact that the CEGB considers a downwind sector out to 3 km (1.75 miles) as the maximum that need be planned for evacuation in the case of a Magnox reactor, while for an AGR the distance is 1 km (0.5 miles). Planning for such evacuation needs to be flexible as, if the 1 km line happened to go through a housing area, it would be very difficult to explain to residents why one side of a street was to be evacuated but not the other, simply because it lay a few metres outside the 1 km radius. In the case of Lancashire, a working party of emergency services and local and other authorities recognised a significant problem in this regard as the Heysham A and Heysham B AGRs are located in a built-up area. They have therefore extended their evacuation area out to a geographical 1 km (0.5 miles) to account for blocks of population. A further realistic measure taken is to acknowledge that, as at TMI, many people may decide to evacuate themselves regardless of the authorities. The Lancashire plan therefore provides temporary shelter for 10 000 evacuees and is being developed to cope with a large scale 'self-evacuation'.

The plan accepts that it is not going to be possible to turn back such people, therefore they should be allowed to go. However, control and organisation are essential if panic is not to break out leading to chaos on the roads. The police have therefore had to prepare route plans to cater for this event. Furthermore, documentation of as many people as possible is needed to reunite separated families and provide information for anxious relatives.

Consideration of Fig. 15.1 demonstrates how the plan will work. Evacuees from the official evacuation zone will be transferred to Ryelands House in Lancaster via one of the two routes shown, depending on conditions at the time, where registration and sorting will take place. Surrounding schools that can provide accommodation for 10 000 people have been earmarked. If people do not have their own transport, buses will be used to carry out the evacuation of the officially recognised risk zone. Arrangements have also been made to remove sick and frail elderly persons from this area. Establishment of traffic control and a one-way system will be the responsibility of the police. This is crucial as it leaves a route free for the emergency services to use to access the Heysham area.

The plan envisages that self-evacuating people from outside the immediate area of the power station will be directed on to the evacuation route and on to Carnforth and Lancaster where registration will take place. After that, they will be free to leave the area to

199

travel to the location they have chosen.

The OSC for an incident at Heysham is located in Lancaster. Senior personnel of the emergency services and local and other authorities would attend the OSC and be in touch with their respective HQs. The advantage of this is that it frees communications in the immediate vicinity of the power station and permits personnel there to get on with the priority tasks.

Emergency service staff need to be included in the detailed planning in order for such plans to be the best possible, and to have the maximum chance of working, all services must have had input.

One final observation concerns the transport of nuclear fuel flasks by rail. In 1984, the CEGB bought a diesel locomotive and three carriages from British Rail (BR). As an experiment they arranged for the locomotive and three carriages to be accelerated up to 160 k.p.h. (100 m.p.h.) before hitting the nuclear fuel flask. The result was that the locomotive was totally wrecked, but the flask remained intact. This demonstration indicates the low probability of a radioactive leak occurring from a flask in a transit accident. Regular exercises are held between the CEGB, BR, and the emergency services covering various contingencies that could arise.

If there is a problem with a flask accident, it concerns the possible location of the incident. Power stations represent fixed localities that can be well protected from a security point of view and permit detailed contingency planning. However, a flask in transit is mobile, and while BR are able to plot its exact position, the train is more vulnerable to attack than a power station. It is also apparent that terrorists would find the containment of a flask easier to breach than a reactor. If a serious accident did occur, it could happen anywhere along the track. Evacuation plans would therefore have to be much more flexible to cope with any eventuality. Once again, there is the dilemma that as the probability of a serious accident becomes extremely remote, the implications of that accident become more and more serious. How much time and effort should emergency services put into developing plans to cope with a major nuclear fuel flask breach? For example, if a hospital lies within a few kilometres of a main railway line transporting spent fuel to Sellafield, could the hospital be evacuated in a few hours, or, as plans envisage for many American hospitals in the aftermath of TMI, effectively go into a state of siege while the radioactive cloud blows over?

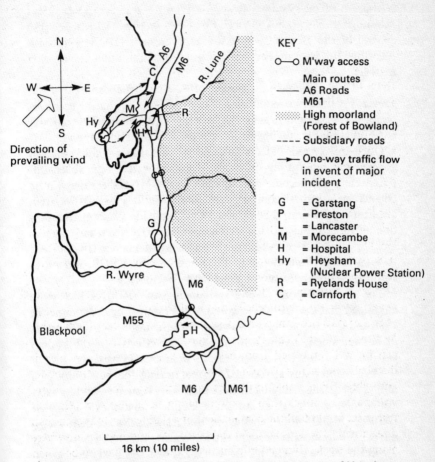

KEY

○——○ M'way access

Main routes
—— A6 Roads
M61

░░░ High moorland
(Forest of Bowland)

- - - - Subsidiary roads

——➤ One-way traffic flow
in event of major
incident

G = Garstang
P = Preston
L = Lancaster
M = Morecambe
H = Hospital
Hy = Heysham
(Nuclear Power Station)
R = Ryelands House
C = Carnforth

Direction of
prevailing wind

16 km (10 miles)

Fig. 15.1 Map showing location and surrounding area of Heysham Nuclear Power Station.

Nuclear accidents in Europe

There was widespread concern amongst the general public after Chernobyl about delays in publicising radiation levels in the UK. In this period it took the EPO in at least one major county two days to get a telephone call through to the NRPB, a very unsatisfactory state of affairs.

In response to this incident the government have announced the setting up of the National Response Plan for Radioactive Incident Monitoring Network (RIMNET). This system falls under the control of the Department of the Environment (DOE) who will, according to government, set up a national radiation monitoring network.

The DOE have proposed a list of 80 sites which will carry out gamma ray dose rate monitoring. There will also be routine monitoring of rainwater and primary water supply at some of these sites. A back up system involving airborne monitoring is also planned.

Once this system detects an incident overseas a whole range of government monitoring on crops, drinking water, vegetables, imports, etc., will become operational. The RIMNET results will be collated in a central computer in London with a back up system duplicating the central computer located outside London. In addition to monitoring radiation effects on the UK from an overseas incident, this system will permit monitoring of a major UK incident at long range from the site. Provision by the CEGB and other authorities already exists for short range monitoring.

The DOE Report (1988) announcing the RIMNET scheme envisaged that the first phase would be operational by the summer of 1988 and the second phase two years after the first. Such a scheme is to be welcomed, but it will only be fully effective if the system permits rapid dissemination of results to interested parties.

This chapter was introduced by mentioning the possibility of a military accident involving nuclear materials. If such an accident did not involve a nuclear explosion, it is likely that the Ministry of Defence (MOD) would endeavour to deal with the accident themselves. While security matters are important, it is to be hoped that the health of the general public would not be a secondary consideration to security, and that the MOD would be forthcoming and cooperative with the civilian services.

Going one step beyond such a scenario, we are left to contemplate the possibility of the accidental detonation of a nuclear warhead in peacetime. The consequences of such an event would be nationwide and would require the mobilisation of the whole of government's resources to try and mitigate the catastrophic effects of such an explosion. International aid would be required as the effects of a single medium sized warhead would be far greater than the NHS could cope with (BMA, 1983; RCN, 1983). It is worth asking what plans the government has to coordinate resources on a national scale to deal with such a disaster. Beyond this point, we are looking into the awful abyss of nuclear war from which there is no way back.

Conclusion

There is a major dilemma inherent in nuclear accident planning which may be stated as follows; what is the worst credible accident it is worth planning for as opposed to the worst possible accident that might happen? We can be confident that Chernobyl or TMI will not happen in the UK and that British reactors are as safe as they can be. Greater openness on the part of the nuclear industry is to be welcomed, as is the improved operational record of BNFL Sellafield. But when all is said, we must be prudent and have plans to cope with the remote possibility of a major incident, plans that are realistic and flexible and, crucially, equally well known to *all* the emergency services.

References

Breo, D. L. (1979). Nuclear scare tests hospital disaster plan. *Journal of the American Association*, May, 33–6.

British Medical Association. (1983). *The Medical Effects of Nuclear War.* John Wiley, Chichester.

Dace, M. (1987). *Radiation and Health.* Medical Campaign Against Nuclear Weapons, London.

Department of Environment. (1988). *Nuclear Accidents Overseas.* HMSO, London.

Gittis, J. H. (1987). The Chernobyl accident and its consequences. *Atom*, United Kingdom Atomic Energy Authority.

Griffiths, R. (1978). Reactor accidents and the environment. *Atom*, United Kingdom Atomic Energy Authority.

Lesher, D., and Bomberger, A. (1979). Experience at Three Mile Island. *American Journal of Nursing*. August, 1402–8

National Radiation Protection Board. (1981). *Specifications in Relation to Emergency Reference Levels.* HMSO, London.

Royal College of Nursing. (1983). *Nuclear War, Civil Defence and the Implications for Nursing.* Royal College of Nursing, London.

16

A man and a gun: the Hungerford massacre, 1987
Anne Eggleton

Setting the scene

Wednesday, 19 August 1987, began as an average quiet day. In the morning the casualty department at Princess Margaret Hospital, Swindon, Wiltshire, had dealt with the usual casualty patients; cut fingers, road traffic accidents (none serious) and sprained ankles. It was to become evident to us all that the casualty staff maxim 'however a shift begins it is not always how it finishes' is very true.

The incident begins

Sometime between 11.00 hours and midday on 19 August, Michael Ryan shot and killed a woman in Savernake Forest, near Marlborough, Wiltshire, leaving her two small children to wander alone in the forest.

He then made his way by car along the main Marlborough to Hungerford road, stopping to refuel the car at a garage at Froxfield, on the Wiltshire/Berkshire border.

After refuelling he took a shot at the woman cashier, luckily missing her. He then continued on to his home town of Hungerford. For those who do not know Hungerford, it is a small market town in Berkshire, some 22 km (14 miles) to the east of Swindon, and this is where Michael Ryan was to become responsible for the worst criminal massacre in the history of the British Isles.

Our involvement

At 13.15 hours a call was received from Berkshire Ambulance Control saying that there had been an incident in Hungerford. It appeared that a person believed to be a mentally disturbed male had shot and injured four people.

At this time, we had no idea of exactly what was going on as the area is a radio black spot. Approximately ten minutes later we had a telephone call from Wiltshire Ambulance Control to say that four casualties were on their way to us from Hungerford and that they were believed to be seriously injured. The initial call that was received by Berkshire Ambulance Control was believed to be a road traffic accident and as they were busy they asked Wiltshire Ambulance Control for assistance. It was not until the Wiltshire crew arrived at the scene that they realised that the man had been shot in the neck. They notified their control that this did not appear to be a normal incident, and how right they were!

Organisation within the department

The resuscitation room and two theatres in the A&E department were prepared and the on call team alerted. Intravenous infusions were set up and trollies prepared for chest drain procedures and major abdominal and head injuries. Although the staff worked with great efficiency and speed to prepare for these patients, we were still unsure exactly what to expect, so the atmosphere in the department was slightly tense and subdued.

The service manager for the trauma unit was informed, as per hospital instructions, as was the senior nurse coming on duty for the late shift.

It was decided to organise the department so that teams were allocated patients after initial assessment and triage had taken place at the ambulance receiving point. The triage was done by an extremely experienced senior A&E nurse, as the senior doctor was unavailable at that time due to another emergency that had occurred earlier. The teams included a senior house officer (SHO), casualty or orthopaedic, an A&E trained nurse, and a junior nurse. These teams were added to as the need arose and, as other specialists were informed of the incident, teams were then made up using SHOs and registrars from other specialities. As the incident progressed, some teams required more medical and nursing staff depending on the degree of injury that the patients had suffered. As patients were admitted via the triage point, they were documented and allocated emergency numbers to facilitate the taking of blood specimens, etc., until their identity could be verified. Portering services were mustered so that the approach to the hospital was kept as clear as possible, as we were now approaching peak visiting time. As I awaited the arrival of the first ambulance, I was extremely surprised to see a photographer and reporter from the local press directly opposite to where the ambulances would pull in and unload! An administration officer was informed and he asked them to move from this area and they quickly complied. As became apparent, this was nothing compared to the legions of international press and media that arrived very rapidly!

We were still suffering from communication problems and as yet had very little information although the administration control centre that had been set up was trying very hard to gain further information for us.

When the first vehicle arrived, it contained two seriously injured patients. They were assessed and allocated to areas within the department. We were fortunate that the situation had arisen at the changeover period in the shifts so that I also had a sister on duty with me who could help coordinate the organisation of the department.

The serious condition of the patients was quite a shock, and it is an experience that I hope is never repeated in my career or in this country again. I think in our minds we were expecting injuries similar to those caused by an air rifle, but these were unlike any injuries that we have come across before. They may be familiar to people who live and work in areas of civil unrest, but even then not in such a large number of patients, or in such a short period of time. The shots appeared to have been fired with reasonable accuracy and, although the entry wound only appeared small, the exit wounds were at times extremely large and had caused multiple trauma and soft tissue injury.

The first patients were taken into the department, together with one of the ambulance crew who, it transpired, had come under fire whilst going to the aid of one of the casualties and had been injured by broken glass from the ambulance windscreen. She, luckily, was not seriously injured, but the patients that she brought in were.

The patients were quickly assessed and the resuscitation measures required were administered. Speed became the essence as information was still scanty about the numbers and conditions of the casualties that we would still receive. The only additional information that we received from the scene was that the incident was still in progress and to expect further seriously injured casualties, numbers unknown, but there had been a number of fatalities.

The next ambulance seemed to arrive very rapidly after the first and contained two severely injured people. One had received shots to the neck and multiple shots to the abdomen, the other had received shots to the abdomen and femur which had caused severe vascular damage. Both patients were extremely shocked and needed immediate operative treatment. Senior surgical and anaesthetic staff were now assisting in the department. Routine theatre lists were cancell:d to facilitate the urgent operative treatment that was required by some of the casualties. Emergency treatments were also carried out in the department, e.g., tracheostomy and Burr holes, as there was not time to get these patients to theatre due to the seriousness of their condition.

By now, the potential magnitude of the incident was becoming clearer. An operations incident control point was set up close to the department in a room specifically designated for this purpose. This control point was manned by the unit managers and the police to coordinate the hospital reaction to the incident, and also to deal with the press and media enquiries which were becoming more numerous by the minute. Support people were called upon to deal with the relatives, and extra clerical staff were required to help with the documentation of the patients and to list and take charge of patients' property. A separate telephone number was provided by the police as a casualty information bureau and this number was publicised via the media. However, this did not stop the pressure of calls from the press all wanting updated information. This made it very important to keep the records as up-to-date as possible regarding identification of patients and condition reports. This was not only for the press, but, more importantly, for the relatives that were telephoning for information as well.

By this time, the resuscitation room (two bays), the two A&E theatres, and the major injury cubicles were full so the back up plan of putting less injured patients into the 11 bedded observation ward was put into operation. While the Hungerford massacre was in progress, the department was still open for normal casualties. Major casualties were assessed and seen in priority order. Minor casualties were informed that there was a major incident, their injuries were assessed, and they were told that there would be a long wait. Many in fact elected to go home and return later. Not surprisingly, when the news was broadcast on the media, the minor injury cases attending became minimal until the next morning.

During the next six hours time itself became unimportant. Although it had been decided not to declare this a major incident, extra staff had been drafted into areas that required them, and a central pool of staff was established nearby so that assistance could be dispatched rapidly should the need arise. Another communication factor that caused a small problem was that, following a request to a local nursing agency for extra ICU nurses to work that night, the local radio station broadcast a request for any nurses to telephone the hospital urgently. Consequently, we were inundated with nurses telephoning in to offer their services. This was done with very good intention, but it did add to the communication chaos for a while. However, enough staff were found for the ICU that night, which was a satisfactory outcome to the problem.

The staff themselves worked quietly and professionally in every sense of the word. Although staff had been on duty for a period of ten hours or more, no one complained and, though the atmosphere of the department seemed almost electric, there was a great feeling of teamwork from the highest to the lowest member of staff. In a way, this provided a means of support for all. However, some staff were beginning to show signs of stress, most noticeable by uncharacteristic comments and the unwillingness to go for a refreshment break. This had to be handled gently but firmly as patients were still arriving and we had no idea how much longer the incident was going to go on as information from the scene was still scanty. Eventually an ambulance liaison officer arrived and set up a telephone link with the ambulance control. From then on, information on exactly what was going on became available more quickly.

After 13 patients had been received we had reached saturation point with regard to theatre time as all the patients required prompt surgical attention and available ICU beds. On the decision of the senior medical staff, a local Royal Air Force (RAF) hospital, who had previously been alerted, was asked if they could assist. They agreed to take the next six casualties (three major, three minor) but, as the situation turned out, the scene was apparently shut down and they were only required to take two patients. One of the patients had been assessed and then after initial treatment had been carried out was transferred to the RAF hospital for further evaluation and admission. The incident was terminated at approximately 18.00

hours, but we were not stood down until 19.45 hours as there was a possibility that there would be more survivors, but, sadly this was not the case. It was also a possibility that the gunman would be brought in. This, in fact, did not happen. However, thought had to be given to this possibility, which would have increased the stress put on the staff, and may have proved difficult for the relatives to cope with. The relatives that had arrived at the hospital were allocated specific rooms a little way from the actual department where they were cared for by members of the hospital chaplains department and the support services. Accommodation was arranged for relatives of the critically ill so that they would be nearby.

Throughout the whole incident, we never officially reached major incident status, but one of the lessons learned from the debrief the next day is that some sort of policy would be required to cope with a mini incident, e.g., ten patients or less depending on the type of incident and the injuries to patients that were involved. Following this debrief, the hospital's Major Incident Plan was rewritten, taking this point into account.

The staff of all types and disciplines that were on duty that day worked efficiently and deserve great credit for the way the whole incident was handled. However, another lesson that was learnt was that support and counselling needed to be available, not only for the patients, but for the staff involved as well. This was provided by a consultant psychiatrist and social workers on an unofficial basis. Staff were encouraged to say how they felt and this counselling was carried on for as long as the people involved felt they needed it.

The other major problem that we as a profession are not used to dealing with is the sheer volume of interest that this type of incident generates to the press and media. Although the press were very cooperative, the large numbers of press and media that were on the hospital site for several days meant that one could not walk freely in the hospital grounds without being accosted by some of them. This can be unnerving, as can giving an interview for national television and press. It is definitely not just one camera and microphone as one tends to think in one's naivity!

It is a day that nobody will forget, but it is one that should be remembered for good teamwork from all disciplines of staff in a difficult and unique incident.

On a personal note, I opened the doors of one of the ambulances to find a good friend (an ambulanceman who my husband had trained with and who lives and works in Hungerford and who I have known for ten years) shot through the knee. I was also aware that my husband (who is an ambulanceman) was attending at the scene and I had no contact with him until he came home that night. Professionalism and the need to keep calm for the sake of other staff kept me going. This is a situation that anyone who works in an A&E department must face every day.

17

Conclusion: the future of disaster planning in the United Kingdom

It is hoped that this book will have given food for thought, both in terms of the theory of what should happen which has been discussed in the first part, and the experiences of what actually has happened described in the second part. Whether the reader be based in the community as a member of the emergency services, or in hospital, she/he should look to their own contingency plans and ask whether in the light of what they have read, they feel confident that those plans are the best that could be laid for a major disaster.

Several themes run through the accounts of the various disasters of the last few years, and this book will conclude by discussing some of them.

The mobile team

The theory of what the mobile team should be able to achieve has been well described in Chapter 5. However, the accounts given here show that such a team has rarely functioned in the way envisaged. The Regent's Park bombing saw the mobile team unable to find its doctors, setting off with three out of four nurses who had no idea of what they were supposed to do, and upon arrival at the scene finding they were not required. The Abbeystead explosion saw the team immobilised by a lack of ambulance transport and unable to get to the scene unless they used their own vehicles. Other accounts speak of there being nothing the team could do when they arrived.

The development of advanced life-saving skills such as intubation and airway management, intravenous infusion techniques, etc., among ambulance personnel means that among the first wave of rescuers on site, there are personnel with many of the medical skills required. This clearly reduces the dependence of the rescue services upon hospital staff.

A second factor is the geography of the UK. We live in a small country with, usually, good communications. Consequently, it is often possible for the ambulance service to evacuate most of the casualties to the hospital before hospital staff can reach the scene. The medical team may arrive only to help with the body count.

If these two factors are combined with poor organisation and training, it is not surprising that hospital mobile teams appear to have had little beneficial effect in many situations. Are such teams therefore worth persevering with as part of disaster planning?

There is a need to logically think through the role of the mobile team and to define exactly what it is to achieve. A detailed analysis of disasters over the last decade should be carried out to provide a critical evaluation of the effectiveness of such teams. In the light of such a rigorous analysis, it may be possible to define situations when a team would be of value and, therefore, who should belong to the team, what training and equipment is needed, and whether a team should be based on every A&E unit. It might be thought better to have a subregional team covering several health authorities which would be available to intervene in specific situations such as casualty entrapment. By limiting the number of teams in this way, it may be possible to give them the necessary resources of equipment and experience that are required. Geographical factors will also play a major role, as the needs in London may be very different from a mountainous area such as Cumbria or a remote county such as Cornwall.

Communications

The various examples discussed here have all highlighted the problem of communication, with hospital switchboards being a principal log jam. Hospitals must find ways of bypassing their switchboards, including giving A&E units direct access to outside lines.

Communication between hospitals and the emergency services has been another problem. Various solutions have been described in this book, all of which have evolved locally. When an aeroplane catches fire on take off at an international airport it should be expected that the local A&E unit would be told what was happening and to activate their disaster plan. This did not happen at Manchester. When a dangerously armed man is shooting everybody that he sees, somebody should tell the A&E unit what is going on. Nobody did at Swindon for many hours.

Is it acceptable that hospital A&E units should have to listen to the radio to find out what is happening in major disaster situations?

There is an urgent need for an investigation into how hospital A&E units communicate with the emergency services in the field during a disaster as this is a key weakness. If a national study were carried out, it should be possible to lay down guidelines for good practice based on the experience that has been gained the hard way in real disaster situations.

Transport

A feature of rescue work in other European countries is the use of helicopters, not only in mountainous remote areas, but also in densely inhabited and congested urban areas. A recent example involved the use of helicopters to evacuate casualties from the wreckage of the trains that crashed at a main line station in Paris. Given the dreadful state of the centre of London and some other large cities, would helicopters not provide a more rapid means of transport? Anyone who has ever gone to an area such as Cornwall for their summer holidays might also ponder the effectiveness of helicopters to airlift casualties from a major incident in rural areas, compared to ambulances labouring their way through the traffic jams.

Such a development would be expensive of course, but it should be remembered that a 'heliambulance service' would be available all the year round to carry urgent, non-disaster cases and could cover a very wide area. It would also fit into a subregional major trauma scheme where one hospital might provide the expertise in multi-trauma management for a catchment covering several health authorities.

Burns

A major theme running through the disasters of the last few years has been the high incidence of burn injury. We live in a very inflammable world whether it be the materials used in constructing the urban environment of the late twentieth century, or the fuels that make motor, air and rail transport possible. The Piper Alpha oil rig disaster in the North Sea is the most recent example of such a trend with the majority of the survivors suffering severe burns, as they did at Abbeystead, the M6 and M61 crashes, Bradford, Manchester Airport and Kings Cross St Pancras.

Hospitals must recognise that there is a high probability of receiving substantial numbers of burns casualties from a major incident. At present, serious burns cases are frequently managed in regional units, with the result that experience of burns may be limited in many hospitals. Wise precautions would therefore include an increase in the quantities of burns dressings held in stock for major incidents, along with a revision of the amounts and types of IV fluids available. Nursing staff who are to be responsible for the running of the casualty reception ward should have an up-to-date knowledge of burns management; in-service training is therefore required. The same comment also applies to medical staff.

In the aftermath of the Piper Alpha tragedy there have been calls for the setting up of a national system to mobilise resources to look after the large number of burns cases that are generated by a major disaster. Given the highly specialised care burns casualties need and the fact that such expertise tends to be concentrated in only one specialist unit per region, a national burns team approach seems long overdue and is to be strongly advocated.

Such a system could send doctors and nurses with the necessary experience to the hospitals where they are most needed for as long as they are needed. By spreading the load nationally, it should make the burden acceptable to any one unit. There are very strong psychological reasons for keeping the casualties together rather than splitting them up around the country, in addition to the physical reasons connected with whether they are fit enough to travel.

Psychological welfare

It is only in the last few years that there has been an awareness of the psychological impact of disasters upon survivors and rescuers. This is an area that demands urgent research for, apart from anything else, it might explain the reluctance of many personnel to take disaster planning seriously. Is it a form of coping by denial, the 'it will never happen here' mentality?

Plans for the future might have a more rational basis if we had insights into how and why people behave the way they do at a disaster. Care for the survivors would also be more complete if it recognised their long-term psychological needs, as would care for the staff who have to deal with disaster as part of their everyday job.

Central planning and coordination

At the moment, the UK seems to have no coordinated strategy for coping with major disaster. Each health authority works under broad guidelines, but very much on its own. There are Home Office guidelines and circulars which cover local authorities and the police. The picture is a very disjointed one with no central control.

There is little facility for learning from other people's experience, little sharing of knowledge gained the hard way when disaster has occurred. Consequently, authorities are always in danger of wasting time and resources reinventing the wheel in dealing with problems. More worrying is the fact that they may not even be aware that they have a problem at all until the event happens.

The need is for government to review disaster procedure and pick out the good practice from the bad, the lessons learned from the mistakes made. Only by evaluating what has gone before can we plan for the future. The time has come therefore for a major initiative to carry out a disaster audit, the outcome of which should be recommendations covering areas such as communication between the different services, the role of mobile hospital teams, the use of alternative forms of transport to the traditional ambulance, sub-regional and national teams of clinical experts, and the psychological welfare of survivors, rescuers, and the families of the casualties.

It may be more appropriate if research into these areas was commissioned by the government but carried out by an independent body such as an appropriate university department, or a specially set up commission of inquiry. The government would be doing the citizens of this country a great service by taking such an initiative, and an even greater service by setting up a central government office with total responsibility for coordinating disaster planning and action to implement its recommendations.

We can no longer muddle through in the time-honoured way. Disasters affect too many people's lives in too many ways to rely on the present well-intentioned but inevitably disjointed and at times, by comparison with other countries, amateurish system.

Postscript: Lockerbie

On 21 December 1988, as this book was going to press, Pan Am flight 103 out of Heathrow became the victim of a terrorist bomb and the UK had one of its worst disasters ever to contend with. The following postscript sets out the main events and what lessons may be learned from them, as far as it is possible to say at this early stage.

The plane in question, a Boeing 747 jumbo jet, took off at 18.25, destination New York. On board were 255 adults and 4 children, most of the passengers were American and many of the rest were British, flying to the USA for Christmas. The plane flew up over the Midlands climbing to 7620 metres (25 000 feet) over Leicestershire, passing over Derby having levelled out at 8530 metres (28 000 feet), on past Manchester and after climbing to 9450 metres (31 000 feet) it flew over Lake Windermere in Cumbria. At 19.01 hours the captain asked Shannon Air Traffic Control for a routing out over the Atlantic Ocean. Two minutes later, when the plane was 32 km (20 miles) north west of Carlisle, Prestwick Air Traffic Control checked to see if the captain had contacted Shannon, there was no reply. Horrified controllers at Prestwick watched the plane's radar blip on their screens disappear to be replaced by a group of smaller blips which gradually faded from the screen. A bomb in the forward luggage hold had detonated ripping the plane apart in midair.

It took approximately four minutes for the blazing wreckage to reach the ground. The strong westerly winds scattered debris over a hundred square miles, while mailsacks and documents were retrieved some 64 km (40 miles) downwind of Lockerbie in Northumbria.

A large amount of the plane wreckage hit the small town of Lockerbie, including a massive fireball of blazing aviation fuel. One section of the plane grazed the main A74 trunk road between Carlisle and Glasgow excavating a 12 metre (40 feet) deep crater on impact in a quiet residential street, Sherwood Crescent. The effect of the impact and blazing fuel was devastating. Two houses completely vanished and 10 more were damaged beyond repair. The bodies of those inside had ceased to exist, they had been vapourised by the crash. It was some days before the police could feel confident about the number of fatalities on the ground, the final figure was 11. Three burnt-out vehicles were left stranded on the A74; it was several days before all the people in them could be accounted for, it appeared they had all survived.

Large sections of the plane cleared the main Glasgow to London railway line and ploughed into the Rosebank Crescent area of the town. Many houses were wrecked here but fortunately this area was spared the burning aviation fuel that caused so much devastation in Sherwood Crescent. In total some 200 people were left homeless by the crash. This area contained the greatest concentration of bodies, some 60 being found on the nearby golf course. The cockpit of the plane came to earth some 5 km (3 miles) away close to Tundergarth Parish Church.

Eyewitness accounts told of the sky appearing to rain metal and flame, and a great rumbling and roaring sound was described by several survivors. At least one person is reported as thinking a nuclear bomb had been dropped on the town. A common theme running through survivor's tales is of chaos and people running to their homes immediately, searching for their families. It has to be remembered that this all happened in the dark with no prior warning.

Royal Air Force (RAF) rescue helicopters were scrambled immediately, and two mountain rescue teams and a coastguard team made their way in the dark to the hills and moors around Lockerbie. The small civilian airport at Carlisle became a refuelling base for the helicopters which were to become a distinctive part of the whole operation in the days and weeks that followed. An initial incident control was set up at Lockerbie Police Station with improvised helicopter landing facilities.

Despite the scale of the disaster, the National Health Service (NHS) was to have little involvement in the events that followed, and only five people needed treatment in hospital, which was provided at Dumfries. This was an example of a massive disaster which produced few surviving injured casualties for the ambulance

217

and hospital services, although this could not have been apparent until well into the night. The Cumberland Infirmary in Carlisle went on stand-by as soon as news of the incident broke, but stood down about an hour later. The nearest major hospital facilities to the scene of the disaster were all 24 to 32 km (15 to 20 miles) away.

Daylight on 22 December brought home to many the scale of the disaster. By this stage it was apparent that a major search and recovery operation had to take place aimed at finding the bodies of the dead and the wreckage of the plane so that investigation into the cause of the disaster could begin. This operation was hindered by sightseers who caused considerable traffic obstruction around the area, and even many days later there was dangerous congestion on the busy A74 trunk road as curious drivers slowed down from their normal speeds to look out over the scene of the crash.

It was clear at this stage that it was not a midair collision that had caused the crash, therefore, either a major structural failure or a bomb were the likely causes.

The search and recovery operation had at its peak 1000 men, including troops from the Gordon Highlanders and a large RAF contingent flying endless helicopter sorties throughout the short daylight hours. Debris from the plane and the bodies of the casualties were in this way located and transported back to Lockerbie where the town hall had become a temporary mortuary. As a mark of respect the Christmas tree and lights were taken down from the town hall roof.

Reports spoke of the strong community spirit in the town over the Christmas period as townspeople helped the servicemen and police with, amongst other things, the traditional British tea and biscuits. There was a strong feeling emerging amongst the local population of wanting to get away from the media and the public gaze because they found it intrusive and tiresome, and also local people realised they had a huge task in grieving for the dead and rebuilding normality in the damaged parts of the town. Around this time, the families of the casualties began to arrive from the USA to see the area where the crash had happened and to mourn their dead.

We have seen earlier in the book how the bereaved need to fully accept the death of their loved ones before the work of grief and recovery can commence. Actually seeing the body is a key part of that process, which was one very important reason to try and recover every single body if possible. A second reason was forensic. If pieces of metal and debris were found imbedded in the bodies of the dead, this would point towards a bomb blast as the likely cause. Such evidence was accumulating by 27 December when 240 bodies had been recovered.

The wreckage of the plane is clearly crucial in determining the cause of the disaster. An explosion on board would have left tell-tale traces of high velocity fragments impacting not only against humans, but also against the material of the plane itself. By 27 December, not only had such evidence been found with regard to the bodies of the dead, but it was reported that suitcases had been found which had been ripped by flying metal fragments and also that the recovered plastic lining of the cargo hold showed heat damage consistent with a flash from a bomb.

The following day, it was announced that scientists from the Royal Armaments Research and Development Establishment had found traces of plastic explosives on sections of a metal pallet from the forward cargo hold. This confirmation of a terrorist bombing brought the incident firmly within the field of the British security services and the American Federal Bureau of Investigation (FBI). Such agencies had to be accommodated alongside the local police, Ministry of Defence experts, the RAF and Army, the Scotland Yard Anti-Terrorist Squad, and a 30-strong contingent from the Air Accident Investigation Branch of the Department of Transport. It can be seen that a large incident control is essential in a disaster of this scale, involving as it does so many different agencies. In this case the Lockerbie Academy was used.

By New Year's Eve a major support and counselling effort was in full swing involving a team of 70 social workers based in a caravan. They were helping people on the telephone, supporting the search parties and aiding the bereaved relatives, mostly from the USA. The relatives all spoke of how coming to Lockerbie had helped them come to terms with their loss. Lessons learned by social workers after the Piper Alpha fire, King's Cross and in Bradford were now being put into practice to help in Lockerbie. It was the sheer volume of the problems that made it so different from the normal support and counselling of everyday social work.

The proximity of Christmas and all that it entails undoubtedly added a unique dimension to this tragedy. All the ideals of love and peace lay scattered across the bleak mid-winter hills of southern Scotland in a trail of wreckage and bodies. Searchers spoke of following a line of wreckage to find two neatly wrapped Christmas puddings, then a teddy bear, and then the body of its young owner. Christmas gifts littered the hills along with the bodies of those who were taking them home to families they would never see again. Many members of the search parties who worked over these hills day after day must have suffered great emotional trauma at finds such as these, as must the farmer who on hearing the explosion and seeing the sky light up came out of his farmhouse to find his paddock littered in crumpled bodies.

Ronald Fause, writing in *The Times* two days after the crash, spoke of a hard-bitten group of newspaper reporters being given an aerial tour of the disaster scene. They were stunned into silence by the scale of the devastation they witnessed as strong winds blew the coverings off the naked bodies littering the ground, and tangled wreckage lay everywhere. Press reports in the days after the crash continually referred to people visiting the area who described the scene as being far worse than they had ever expected from television news reports.

Two weeks after the crash, the incident control still had a staff of approximately 100 and helicopters were busily ferrying wreckage to Lockerbie. Only 20% of the wreckage had been recovered and 80% located, leaving large parts of the plane still missing. Also missing were the bodies of 20 passengers and 8 of the residents from Sherwood Crescent.

A memorial service for the dead, attended by some 200 relatives from the USA, was held on 4 January 1989. The congregation spilled over into the graveyard of the small church where the service was held. By now 100 bodies had been released for burial, US officials coming to Lockerbie to help with speeding up the process of documentation. The scale of the disaster may be gauged by the fact that the following day, 5 January, the Government announced it was allocating £1 million in aid for the small town of Lockerbie.

This book has contained accounts of disasters, all written some time after the event when there has been time for consideration and analysis. Although this postscript is being written only a few weeks after the crash, there are still lessons that can usefully be learnt. They may be summarised as follows:

1   An aeroplane can crash anywhere. The absence of an airport in an area does not exclude the possibility of an air disaster.

2 In an incident such as this, there are unlikely to be any survivors on the plane. However, there may be many injured on the ground with a large geographical spread, depending on how sections of the plane land. This plane came down over a largely empty, rural district: it might have landed on a major urban area creating a series of separate major incidents as each large section of the plane hit the ground.

3 In the event of a plane (or planes in the event of a midair collision) coming down on an urban area, the scale of what happened at Lockerbie indicates a disaster of horrendous magnitude. Can your area's disaster plans cope with such an event?

4 The need for extensive interdisciplinary communication was demonstrated as such an incident extends far beyond the remit of the fire, police, ambulance and hospital services. An incident control room may have to function over a period of several weeks carrying a staff of up to 100 from a wide range of civilian, military and security agencies.

5 Sightseers caused many problems to the search and rescue services.

6 Hospital staff in Carlisle began telephoning their local hospital as the news broke, jamming the hospital switchboard. A hospital plan usually requires staff to wait until called, and staff must understand that telephoning in like this will only jam the switchboard. This indicates the need for *all* staff to be conversant with their hospital's major incident plan.

7 The casualty bureau telephone numbers used at Lockerbie were inadequate, there were many complaints of jammed lines. It has been reported in the press that the Home Office, the Police and British Telecom are trying to find better ways of improving public access to information after such incidents.

8 The major role of the local authority was demonstrated in this incident, underlining the need for the full involvement of the emergency planning officer's team in planning.

9 The use of helicopters was a major feature of this incident and this is an area that must be developed for the future. In the chaos that might occur if a similar incident happened in an urban area, airlifting casualties might be the only realistic way of getting the seriously injured to hospital quickly enough.

10 Once again the role of fire in causing casualties was shown.

Consider the effects of a cloud of burning aviation fuel hitting an office block or department store in a town centre instead of a small street as at Lockerbie.

11 Rescue personnel need to realise the forensic importance of wreckage and also the needs of the police to protect the scene from theft and looting, as sadly occurred at Lockerbie.

12 The need for counselling and social work support for survivors, the bereaved and rescuers has been vividly demonstrated. It has to be recognised that in allocating resources to cope with major incidents, it is more than a matter of, for example, equipping mobile medical teams. Resources need to be put aside to train staff to provide psychological and social aftercare for perhaps many hundreds of people. The informal links that have grown up in the social services from experiences gained in the aftermath of the Piper Alpha explosion and the Bradford fire, for example, need to be consolidated and organised effectively, with the resources necessary from central government, to provide the care needed over a period of months and years after a disaster.

13 The whole subject of disasters needs to be taken more seriously by the government. Messages of praise for heroics performed by the emergency services and a visit from the Prime Minister are not enough. Research into methods of improving our response to major incidents is desperately needed along with the resources to implement the findings of such an inquiry. A government funded project, carried out independently and as a priority perhaps at a university or a government-appointed committee of inquiry, is urgently needed.

I will conclude by considering two commonly heard excuses for not taking disaster planning seriously, starting with the statement that lightning never strikes in the same place twice, i.e., a fluke like Lockerbie could never happen again. Even as the author was writing this chapter, on the evening of Sunday 8 January 1989, a Boeing 737 from Heathrow took off for Belfast, it ended up sprawled across the M1 motorway with 46 more people dead and another 80 casualties, many seriously injured, needing hospital treatment. Lightning can strike twice, and three and four times. Because a particular type of disaster has happened today, do not think it cannot happen tomorrow.

Finally, consider the 'It can't happen here' approach that introduced this book; an excuse used by some people who should be more involved in disaster planning. It never occurred to me that the first week of 1989 would see the bodies of a student in my own department and her 20 month old daughter, lowered in the same coffin into their grave, killed along with 268 others by a terrorist bomb. Yet that is what happened to Yvonne Owen and her daughter Bryony, buried now in the village of Pendine in Dyfed. It can't happen here? We owe it to the memory of Yvonne Owen and her little daughter, and the hundreds more who have become victims of the 1980s, to believe that it *can* happen here. Such a belief is vital throughout society if we are to prevent disaster ever happening and if we are to have the resources available to cope with the worst if it should occur.

Index

Abbeystead   3, 25, 40, 89
ABC of resuscitation   9, 18, 21,
    74
Aberfan   96
accident proneness   95
action cards   65, 152
AIDS   17
airway   9, 14, 15, 74
alpha radiation   43
Ambubag   34
ambulance service
    responsibilities   53
amputation   30, 32, 33
Armalite rifle   36

BASICS   54, 55, 72
baton rounds   144
bereavement   111
beta radiation   43
Birmingham
    City Football Club   146
    pub bombings   27, 28
Blackpool   89
Blakelock, PC   147
blast
    injury   25, 30
    lung   28
    wave   26
bleeding   19

blood
    grouping on site   76, 178
    loss   18–20
bombs
    effects of   132
    explosive materials   29
    fragmentation   25, 132
    injury patterns   31, 32, 135,
        138
Bophal   186
Bradford
    City Football Club   1, 15, 50
    press facilities   125
    Royal Infirmary, A&E   161
breathing   12, 14, 15, 18, 74
Bristol City Football Club   145
British Nuclear Fuels
    Limited   53, 89, 186
Brixton riots   146
burns
    Abbeystead   177
    airway   15
    Bradford City Football Club
        fire   164
    disaster teams   213
    effects of   37
    first aid   21
    flash   25, 31
    Hyde Park bombing   133

Manchester International
  Airport fire   156
 shock   18
bystanders   94, 109

carbon monoxide   39
cardiopulmonary
  resuscitation   17
carotid pulse   16
casualty
 collection point   82
 collection point Tottenham
   riots   147
 information bureau   51, 123,
   207
CEGB nuclear accident
  plans   194, 195
Chelsea Barracks bombing   131
Chernobyl   43, 189–92
chest
 compression   16
 drainage   35, 75
 injury   14, 33
circulation   15, 75
communications
 Abbeystead   176
 Bradford City Football Club
   fire   163, 165
 Hungerford   205, 208
 inter-service   5, 49, 212
 local authority emergency
   planning office   87
 Manchester International
   Airport fire   158
 Tottenham riots   144
counselling
 Abbeystead   178
 Hungerford   209
 IRA bombings   139
 Manchester International

 Airport fire   159
crush injury   19, 25, 30, 31
CS gas   41

decision making   99
decontamination   45, 52, 196
disaster syndrome   104
District General Manager
  planning role   59
dressings   21, 76
drowning   14
drugs
 Abbeystead   174
 Bradford City Football Club
   fire   167
 Manchester International
   Airport fire   156
 mobile team   77
Dungeness PWR
  (proposed)   194
Dymchurch   194

eardrum rupture   27, 30, 136
earthquake   101
Enniskillin bombing   3, 91, 136
Entonox   77
evacuation and nuclear accidents
 Chernobyl   192
 hospitals   189
 Lancashire   199
 Three Mile Island   188
 UK   194, 198

Falkland Islands War   125
fatigue   98
fear   102
firearms used in riots   142
fire service responsibility   52
flail segment   14, 34
flooding   5, 6, 89

football hooliganism   140, 146
fractures
  femur   19
  rib   14
  signs of   22
  treatment of   23
  tibia   19
fragmentation bombs   25, 34,
    132

gamma radiation   43
Gelofusin   75
grief   111
Guildford pub bombings   29
gunfire aimed at emergency
    personnel   37, 142, 206
gunshot injury   19, 36, 206

Haemaccel   75
haemothorax   14, 33–5, 75
Harrods bombing   137
Havers, Sir Michael QC   131
Heimlich valve   34, 75
helpers   94, 109
helplessness in survivors   103
Heysham A/B nuclear power
    stations   89, 199
high velocity missiles   36
Hiroshima   101
hospital disaster plans
  aims   58, 61
  Preston Royal Hospital   183
  Princess Margaret
      Hospital   205
  Royal Lancaster
      Infirmary   173
  Southampton General
      Hospital   66
  Wythenshawe Hospital   152
hospital managers' role   63

Hungerford
  news coverage   118, 120
  shootings   1, 2, 37, 91, 110
hurricane   6
Hyde Park bombing   132
Hythe   194

information processing   97, 107
interpreters   64
intravenous fluids   75, 76
iodine tablets   46, 197
IRA
  bombs   25, 26, 34, 83, 108
  funerals   124
  UK Prime Minister   89, 128,
      131
Iran-Iraq War casualties   35

Jarrett, Cynthia   140
Joint Incident Room,
    Tottenham riots   144

Kalashnikov AK47 assault
    rifle   36
King's Cross Underground
    fire   91, 123, 125

Lancaster   199
Leeds United Football
    Club   146
Lockerbie air crash   216–23
loss   103
Luton Town Football
    Club   146
Lynmouth   5

Manchester
  International Airport   15
  Royal Infirmary   151

medical organisation for disaster
  plans 62
methane 40
Mill Hill Barracks
  bombing 102
Millwall Football Club 145,
  146
mobile medical team
  Abbeystead 174
  action on site 82
  Bradford City Football Club
    fire 163
  Chernobyl 191
  clothing 80, 148
  equipment 73, 79
  London IRA bombings 134
  personnel 72, 135
  Preston Royal Hospital 184
  role of 4, 55, 71, 211
Moorgate Underground
  disaster 33
mouth-to-mouth
  resuscitation 13, 16
muzzle velocity 35

NAIR 44
narcotic analgesia
  Bradford City Football Club
    fire 167
  mobile medical team 78
National Blood Transfusion
  Service 124, 138
neck injury 11
neutron 43
news
  blackouts 122
  editing 120
newspaper reporting 121
North Middlesex
  Hospital 145, 148

nuclear explosion 193, 202
nursing organisation for
  disaster 62

offshore incidents 57, 83
Omagh bombing 113
Oxford Street bombs 131, 137

pain 19, 22, 24, 78
panic
  Bradford City Football Club
    fire 166
  prevention of by media 122
  psychology of 103,
  radiation incidents 198
petrol bombs 142, 146
Piper Alpha explosion 96, 112,
  214
pneumothorax 14, 33–5, 75
police responsibility 51, 136
post traumatic stress
  disorder 114
press
  Bradford City Football Club
    fire 170
  facilities 57, 126
  Hungerford 206, 209
  Manchester International
    Airport fire 159
  officers 125
  Three Mile Island 188
Preston Royal Hospital,
  A&E 177, 183
Prime Minister 127, 128, 171
Princess Margaret Hospital,
  Swindon 120, 204
Pringle, Sir Stewart 131
Pripyat Hospital, USSR 191
protective clothing 80

psychological
   aftercare   113
   first aid   108

radiation
   casualties   41, 191
   effects of exposure   44, 198
   Emergency Reference
      Levels   198
   monitoring   43, 88, 196
   protection from   45
   sickness syndrome   43, 191
   types   43
   units   42
Radioactive Incident Monitoring
      Network   202
rail transport of nuclear
      waste   200
Regent's Park bombing   132,
      134
Regional Emergency Planning
      Officer, NHS   60
rehearsal of disaster plans   69,
      84
rescuers, psychological
      effects   93
resuscitation   13, 45
riot gear   144
risk assessment   96
Royal Lancaster Infirmary   172
Rye   194

shock
   physiological   18, 20
   psychological   102
shrapnel wounds   133
slings   23
St Luke's Hospital,
      Bradford   165

St Mary's Hospital,
      London   133, 134
St Michael on Wyre   172
St Paul's, Bristol   124
St Stephen's Hospital,
      London   133
Stockport Infirmary   151
stress
   Hungerford   208
   Manchester International
      Airport fire   154
   psychology   105
   Tottenham riots   148
suction   74
survival behaviour   105

tear gas   40
telephone communications
   Abbeystead   177
   Bradford City Football Club
      fire   168, 169
   Harrods bombing   138
   hospital   61, 212
   Hungerford   208
   press   121, 123, 127
   Three Mile Island   188
terrorism and nuclear
      power   195, 200
Thatcher, Mrs   127
Three Mile Island   187
Tottenham riots   6, 82
Tower of London bombing   31
toxic fumes   39
triage   56, 72, 81, 205

unconscious casualties   10, 11,
      14
University College Hospital,
      London   133

ventilators, portable   75
victims, psychology of   93, 113, 114
video   120, 124
Vietnam War casualties   34
vomit   11

Wallace's Rule of Nine   38
Wapping dispute casualties   146
warning of disaster   92, 100
Westminster Hospital   132, 133, 137
Whitehaven   123

Whittington Hospital   145, 148
Withington Hospital   151
Woolwich Barracks bombing   131
World War I casualties   34
World War II casualties   34
wounds   21, 133
Wythenshawe Hospital, A&E   151

X-rays   43

Zeebrugge   8, 91, 119